WII EVASION

Also by Michael Chesbro

The Complete Guide to E-Security:
  Using the Internet and E-mail without Losing Your Privacy

Freeware Encryption and Security Programs:
  Protecting Your Computer and Your Privacy

Privacy for Sale:
  How Big Brother and Others Are Selling Your Private Secrets for Profit

The Privacy Handbook:
  Proven Countermeasures for Combating Threats to Privacy, Security and Personal Freedom

Wilderness Evasion: A Guide to Hiding Out and Eluding Pursuit in Remote Areas
by Michael Chesbro

Copyright © 2002 by Michael Chesbro
ISBN 13: 978-1-58160-365-1
Printed in the United States of America

Published by Paladin Press, a division of
Paladin Enterprises, Inc.
Gunbarrel Tech Center
7077 Winchester Circle
Boulder, Colorado 80301 USA
+1.303.443.7250

Direct inquiries and/or orders to the above address.

PALADIN, PALADIN PRESS, and the "horse head" design are trademarks belonging to Paladin Enterprises and registered in United States Patent and Trademark Office.

All rights reserved. Except for use in a review, no portion of this book may be reproduced in any form without the express written permission of the publisher.

Neither the author nor the publisher assumes any responsibility for the use or misuse of information contained in this book.

Visit our Web site at: www.paladin-press.com

WILDERNESS EVASION

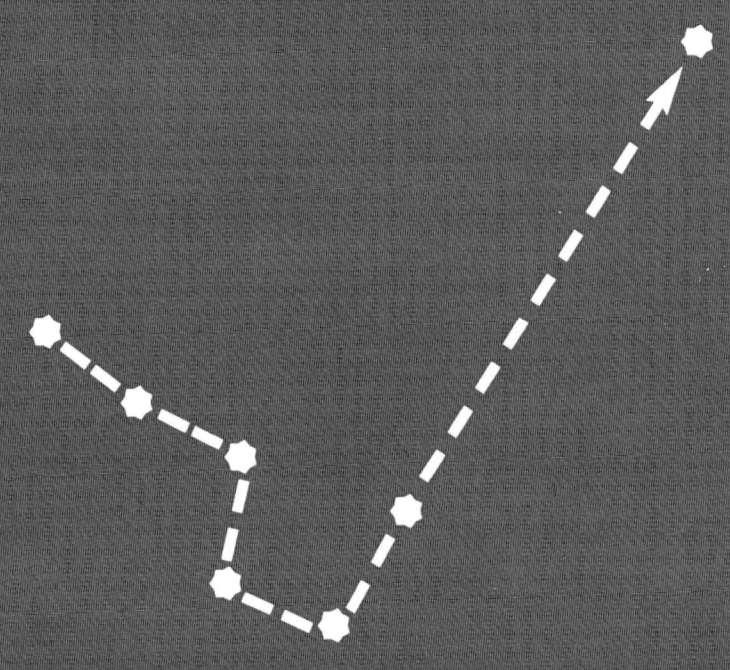

A Guide to Hiding Out and Eluding Pursuit in Remote Areas

Michael Chesbro

PALADIN PRESS • BOULDER, COLORADO

As always . . . for Joni.
There could never be another.

Table of Contents

Introduction	WHY WOULD ANYONE WANT TO HIDE OUT IN THE WILDERNESS?	- 1 -
Chapter 1	DEVELOPING THE PROPER MIND-SET	- 5 -
Chapter 2	BUILDING A GOOD KIT	- 13 -
Chapter 3	CACHES	- 17 -
Chapter 4	GETTING THERE	- 27 -
Chapter 5	RESUPPLY SYSTEMS	- 31 -
Chapter 6	IN AND AROUND TOWN	- 35 -
Chapter 7	EVADING PURSUIT	- 37 -
Chapter 8	COMMUNICATIONS	- 51 -
Chapter 9	COVERT SIGNALS	- 67 -

Chapter 10	NAVIGATION	- 71 -
Chapter 11	FIREARMS FOR SURVIVAL	- 77 -
Chapter 12	PRIMITIVE WEAPONS	- 83 -
Chapter 13	SHELTERS	- 91 -
Chapter 14	FIRE	- 99 -
Chapter 15	CAMOUFLAGE	- 103 -
Chapter 16	FOOD	- 107 -
Chapter 17	WATER	- 121 -
Chapter 18	SURVIVAL MEDICINE	- 125 -
A Final Word		- 149 -
Bibliography and Selected Reading		- 151 -
Resources		- 155 -

Acknowledgments

Although this book is based on my personal studies and training, there are several people who have contributed to my knowledge and experience in these matters and who deserve recognition.

First I want to acknowledge the men of the U.S. Army 1st Special Forces Group (Airborne) with whom it is my great honor and privilege to have served. These men are the true experts in survival and evasion. They are the quiet professionals and the unsung heroes of this great republic.

I would also like to thank Ron and Karen Hood of the Hoods Woods Survival School in Idaho for their outstanding contribution to the field of wilderness survival and personal preparedness. Ron's *Woods Master* videos and Karen's *Cave Cooking* videos are a must for anyone with an interest in survival.

Finally, I would like to thank Olympia Search and Rescue, the trackers, dog search teams, communications center, and medical staff for the opportunity to learn how a professional search team works.

While acknowledging the contributions of all of the people above, I am responsible for the contents of this book, and any shortcomings and errors are mine alone.

—Michael Chesbro
November 2002

Preface

With all the survival books in print and the rash of preparedness books that hit the market prior to Y2K, just why would someone want to write another one? Almost without exception the other survival books make the assumption that you want to be found, that you are making a specific attempt to attract the attention of searchers or rescuers or at the least that you are staying in a particular place with little intention of eluding discovery. Military escape-and-evasion manuals are based on the premise that you will evade the enemy and work your way back to your own lines or be recovered by a combat search-and-rescue team. Military escape-and-evasion techniques have some application in this discussion, but military methods focus on a combat environment with a built-in combat search-and-rescue system and rules of conduct far different from those of daily life.

In this book I look at survival from the viewpoint of staying lost. I discuss methods of hiding out and evading pursuit in the wilderness. In writing this book, I make the assumption that the reader has some degree of outdoor experience. Perhaps you have spent some time backpacking, camping, hunting, or just taking day hikes along established trails. I discuss survival techniques from the point of the evader but leave the most basic survival skills to one or more of the survival books and videos already available. (After all, there are only so many ways to describe how to light a fire with flint and steel.)

Finally, in writing this book, I make the assumption that the reader has moved into a wilderness area to with the intention of evading discovery, and that there is at least a passive attempt by others to locate him. Because you have moved into a wilderness area to deliberately evade pursuit, you should be carrying certain items to aid in your survival and evasion. I discuss those items and how to use them.

Introduction

Why Would Anyone Want to Hide Out in the Wilderness?

Why does anyone pack up and head for parts unknown? Perhaps you are fleeing an abusive relationship, avoiding some overzealous rogue government agency while your attorney sorts out the details, or ducking some criminal element that wants to send over Guido and Lefty to talk about your kneecaps (of course some may view "criminal element" and "government agency" as much the same thing). Even if you are not on someone's 10-most-wanted list, it may be that you simply want to disappear from the view of Big Brother for a while.

There are several books available about establishing new IDs or disappearing and establishing a new life elsewhere. The disadvantage I see to many of these techniques is that they rely on circumstances that may be difficult to arrange, cost much more than many can afford, and tend to leave clues that any good investigator can follow. Finally, these books assume that you will leave all vestiges of your old life behind—which is certainly desirable, but usually requires some transition time between your old life and the new.

The advantage of wilderness evasion is that you leave no clues for investigators: no credit card activity, telephone records, or motor vehicle information. Staking out your old hangouts turns up nothing, and interviews with your friends, acquaintances and co-workers lead to a dead end. Evading in the wilderness is less expensive than other options, and it gives you the option of returning to your life with a plausible reason for being gone—"I spent the summer hiking the Appalachian Trail"— or making the transition to an entirely new life and identity.

Quite simply, "wilderness evasion" allows you to drop off the face of the Earth for a while. In today's "modern society" fewer and fewer people are comfortable in a wilderness environment. The days when so many young men knew how to pitch a tent, build a campfire, hunt wild game, and take care of themselves in the outdoors are gone. Many people can't imagine themselves without television, shopping malls, and an automobile to take them anywhere farther than half a mile.

Anyone comfortable in the wilderness has a distinct advantage if he needs to drop out of sight for a few weeks or a few months.

For people who regularly spend time in the wilderness or live in a remote area, wilderness evasion can serve as a means of self-protection. It takes little effort to find reports in the news of hikers being mugged or campers abducted from their campsites. With the government's current forfeiture policies, marijuana growers and others involved in related activities have moved their operations onto public lands. This may limit the ability of the government to seize their property without trial, but it increases the possibility for people hiking in remote areas to stumble onto marijuana fields and the like. If this happens, there is the possibility of the fields' operators pursuing people who discover such an operation to prevent the fields' being reported.

There are extreme examples of people being hunted in the wilderness. As an example, let's take a look at the case of one

INTRODUCTION

Robert Hansen. Born in Pocahontas, Iowa, in 1939, Hansen was unpopular in his youth and had his first major run-in with the law in 1961 when he was arrested for arson. Six years later, Hansen moved to Anchorage, Alaska, where he opened a bakery, learned to fly, and began to develop a reputation as an avid outdoorsman and hunter. Between 1973 and 1983 Hansen murdered at least 17 women. Kidnapping these women, he would fly them to a remote location outside Anchorage and release them into the wilderness. He would then hunt them down and murder them with knife, bow and arrow, or rifle.

Hansen is not the only killer to hunt people in the wilderness. Between 1989 and 1992, Australia's "Backpack Killer," Ivan Robert Marko Milat, murdered seven backpackers in the Australian outback. Milat kidnapped these backpackers, released them into the wilderness, and then hunted them down, murdering them with a rifle.

Would wilderness evasion skills have allowed the women to escape from Hansen and make their way back to Anchorage or the backpackers to escape Milat and make it to safety? Will having wilderness evasion skills help someone in similar circumstances in the future?

Let's look at the case of Eric Rudolph, the man accused of bombing a Birmingham, Alabama, abortion clinic, and being involved in the 1996 bombing of the Olympic Games in Atlanta, Georgia. He on one of the FBI's "10 Most Wanted," and there is a $1 million reward for his capture.

So why isn't Eric Rudolph in jail? He is a wilderness evader, having escaped arrest by fleeing into North Carolina's Nantahala Mountains. Nobody believes that bombing clinics or athletic events is an admirable activity, and I don't support Rudolph's alleged criminal activity, but he serves as an excellent example of the effectiveness of wilderness evasion. Even with hundreds of searchers called in to pursue Rudolph in the North Carolina mountains, and the million-dollar reward for his capture, Rudolph remains free. Are local residents aiding Rudolph? Probably, but it is his ability to stay hidden in the wilderness that ensures his continued freedom. One man, skilled in wilderness survival and evasion, is extremely difficult to find!

Thus it is my hope that the techniques in this book will benefit those who, while perhaps not evading pursuit in a wilderness area, spend time enjoying the outdoors. A fringe benefit of skill in wilderness evasion is that you leave no trace in the wilderness during the course of normal outdoor activities, such as camping, hiking, or hunting.

CHAPTER 1

Developing the Proper Mind-Set

OK, you've decided that a wilderness getaway may be in your future. If you just grab a blanket and your Boy Scout knife and head for the nearest swamp, chances are that you won't last a week. It is essential that you develop a clear plan of where you're going and what you'll do when you get there.

Depending on where you live, it may be possible to just walk out your back door into the forest and disappear. On the other hand, if you live in a major city, it'll be necessary to have some method of travel to reach a wilderness area in which to evade.

Once you have decided on your initial evasion area, you must learn all that you can about that area. Gather maps of the area, both topographical and any others (such as local road maps) of the area. Can the area be reached by vehicle? How about by horseback? Do tourists or outdoor-adventure types commonly visit the area? Hunters? Learn about the weather patterns in the area. Are there frequent sudden storms, severely cold winters, or drought in the summer?

While studying the area make it a point to learn about plants and animals in the area. What's edible, and what's not? Is there small game or larger that you can use to supplement your diet?

What towns are in the area? How far are they from the specific area in which you plan to stay? What do they have to offer? What are the best routes in and out of the town? Wilderness evasion does not necessarily mean you'll never go near a town. It may even be possible (depending on what type of search you are trying to evade) to make use of campgrounds and some of the facilities offered there.

Along this line, however, ask yourself how far away from any town you need to be to preclude incidental discovery. I have found that moving a distance of two days' hiking time from town (or base areas such as campgrounds and established hiking trails) takes you away from almost all casual hikers and outdoor enthusiasts. If you are within a day's hike of a town you may come across day hikers. On occasion you will find people who hike a day into the woods and set up a camping area, but you almost never see these people making a second day's move into a wilderness area. Two days into the wilderness takes you beyond all but the most avid outdoor enthusiasts and people with a specific purpose (e.g., evasion or searching for you).

EVASION INTELLIGENCE PLAN

As you gather information about your chosen evasion area, assemble it into a notebook. You will make an intelligence package to aid you during your evasion. It will contain the following:

- Evasion intelligence plan format
- General area maps and description
- State map(s)
- Road atlas of surrounding area

DEVELOPING THE PROPER MIND-SET

- Location of airstrips and railroad lines
- Mines, quarries, and dumps
- Specific area topographical maps and charts
- Primary and alternate routes to and from base camp
- Location of water sources (ponds, streams, springs)
- Food source locations (fruit trees, fishing spots, game trails)
- Cache reports
- Communications plan
- Radio frequencies, call signs, and contact times
- Transmission pathways and azimuths
- Local National Oceanic and Atmospheric Administration (NOAA) weather radio frequency
- General broadcast stations receivable from base camp
- Dead drop sites
- Loaded and recovered signal sites
- Supply inventory and resupply plan
- Location of nearest post office or private mail service

As you assemble your evasion intelligence package, you'll want to make it as complete and detailed as possible. There is no such thing as too much detail! You never know what piece of information, though insignificant today, becomes essential tomorrow.

By putting together such a package you develop an in depth knowledge of a given area. This knowledge gives you an essential advantage over any who might attempt to pursue you or search you out. Knowledge builds confidence and quells panic.

NO PANIC

The right mind-set is nothing new. The principles of stealth and evasion in the wilderness have always been the same and will likely remain unchanged for many more generations. In 1736 Maj. Robert Rogers of Rogers' Rangers fame established standing orders for his company of Rangers. Those orders are worth considering by the wilderness evader.

Rogers' Rangers Standing Orders, 1736

1. Don't forget nothing.
2. Have your musket clean as a whistle, hatchet scoured, sixty rounds powder and ball, and be ready to march at a minute's warning.
3. When you're on the march, act the way you would if you were sneaking up on a deer—see the enemy first.
4. Tell the truth about what you see and what you do. There is an army depending on us for correct information. You can lie all you please when you tell other folks about the Rangers, but don't lie to a Ranger or officer.
5. Don't never take a chance you don't have to.
6. When we're on the march we march single file, far enough apart so one round can't go through two men.
7. If we strike swamps or soft ground, we spread out abreast, so it's hard to track us.
8. When we march, we keep moving till dark so as to give the enemy the least possible chance at us.
9. When we camp, half the party stays awake the other half sleeps.
10. If we take prisoners, we keep 'em separate till we have had time to examine them, so they can't cook up a story between 'em.
11. Don't ever march home the same way. Take a different route so you won't be ambushed.
12. No matter whether we travel in big parties or little ones, each party has to keep a scout 20 yards ahead, 20 yards on each flank, and 20 yards in the rear so the main body can't be surprised and wiped out.
13. Every night you'll be told where to meet if surrounded by a superior force.
14. Don't sit down to eat without posting sentries.
15. Don't sleep beyond dawn. Dawn's when the French and Indians attack.
16. Don't cross a river by a regular ford.
17. If somebody's trailing you, make a circle, come back onto your own tracks, and ambush the folks that aim to ambush you.

DEVELOPING THE PROPER MIND-SET

18. Don't stand up when the enemy's coming against you. Kneel down, lie down, hide behind a tree.
19. Let the enemy come till he's almost close enough to touch. Then let him have it and jump out and finish him up with your hatchet.

Although Rogers' Rangers standing orders were intended for a military force, the principles remain valid for the wilderness evader today. Such tactics as number 3 ("When we're on the march, act the way you would if you were sneaking up on a deer—see the enemy first") and number 17 ("If somebody's trailing you, make a circle, come back onto your own tracks, and ambush the folks that aim to ambush you") are directly applicable for our purposes.

If you are forced into an evasion scenario you will find yourself under some degree of stress. Some people work well under stress, others do not, but anyone will fall apart if the stress becomes great enough. By being prepared and developing the proper mind-set you lessen the adverse effects of a stressful situation. The fact that you are reading this book and thinking about the possibility of wilderness evasion is a step in the right direction.

The whole idea is to have the right mind-set during evasion. Don't panic. In the wilderness you will generally have the advantage over your pursuers. Having clear principles established in your mind will keep your thinking focused. Stay focused and don't lose your mind.

Psychological Factors

Once you are in a survival/evasion situation, there are several psychological factors that will affect your ability to survive. You'll experience various emotional reactions, depending on your personality, level of skill, self-confidence, and the environment in which you find yourself. Understanding these psychological factors will help you deal with them, and lessen the effect they'll have on you.

Initial Shock

No matter what causes you to be in a survival situation, it will always be accompanied by some degree of initial shock. This is the result of stress and the disruption of your current life's routine. The extent of the shock will depend on what caused you to be in the situation you find yourself and your level of preparedness to deal with the situation. Resting, evaluating your situation, and formulating a plan of action to deal with the problems at hand can overcome initial shock.

Pain and Injury

In addition to the initial shock of being in a survival situation, you may have to deal with injuries and the pain associated with them. With a planned move into an evasion area, pain and injury are usually limited factors; however, if you are forced into the situation they may be your primary concern. Are you fleeing physical abuse? Did your evasion begin at 2:00 A.M. when a bunch of men wearing face masks, carrying submachine guns, and yelling something you couldn't understand broke through your front door? If you are injured, it is important to treat those injuries as quickly and as completely as possible.

Cold and Heat

Although cold and heat are not themselves psychological factors, they will certainly affect your state of mind. You need to have shelter that protects you from the environment, maintaining a comfortable (or at least reasonable) temperature. This can be as simple as sitting in the shade to stay out of the sun or putting on a jacket to protect you from the cold, or as extensive as securing a shelter in advance and completely stocking it with supplies.

Hunger and Thirst

Hunger and thirst are the body's reaction to lack of food and water. Just because you are hungry does not mean that you are starving to death, but it does mean that you are taking in less food than your body has become accustomed to. In stress situations people often feel the need to eat (having the "munchies") as the body demands higher glucose levels. Thirst, on the other hand, is a clear indicator that your body needs water. You should have at least 2 liters of water per day. Drinking plenty of water (slightly over 2 quarts) and eating regularly go a long way toward reducing stress and limiting adverse psychological factors associated with a survival situation. In the initial stages of the survival situation try to have plenty of water available and some high-energy food.

Fatigue

Proper rest is essential to maintaining a positive psychological state. Even in a survival situation you should plan periods of rest and have a scheduled time for sleep. There is something to be said for the old saying "things will look better after a good night's rest."

After the initial stages of the survival situation have passed, other psychological factors begin to take effect. You have recovered from the initial shock, luckily you've suffered no injuries, and you've had something to eat and drink and even gotten a few hours of sleep. Overall you're in pretty good shape, so just what psychological factors do you have to deal with next?

Fear and Anxiety

Fear and anxiety are part of the initial psychological factors that affect someone in a survival situation, but these factors carry over past the initial stages. As you begin to consider the situation you're in you may experience an increased level of fear and anxiety from both real and imagined threats. If someone is pursuing you with hostile intent, there may be some reason to your fearing his finding you. Fear is best fought with knowledge and self-confidence. You know that you have a problem, but you also know that you can deal with that problem. Bravery is not a lack of fear; it is simply the ability to deal with it. Recognize fear for what it is, tell yourself that you will not let fear defeat you, and it won't!

Boredom and Loneliness

Once you have made your escape into a remote area you may find that you're bored and lonely. Man is a social animal and needs the company of other people. Almost everyone enjoys a little time alone, but when a few days becomes a few weeks or a few months many people have an overwhelming desire for company. Along this same line, once you have made it into the backwoods and established a comfortable shelter with a reasonable supply of food and water, you may become bored. To combat this you should have items available to limit both boredom and loneliness.

Boredom can be avoided by having something to do. This may mean caching a couple of novels that you have been meaning to read. Or maybe instead of novels, you should cache a bunch of pens and paper to allow you to write about your experiences. You may choose to work on your skills with primitive weapons and tools. Loneliness can be a bit more difficult to fight, but maybe you'll be able to visit towns from time to time, or you might have a radio to receive news and entertainment, which can greatly reduce the effects of loneliness.

Depression and Loss of Self-Determination

Finally, you must be aware of the possibility that you may become depressed and generally lose your will to continue. You are in the wilderness; you have left a portion of your life behind, or perhaps you are fighting to get back to it. Depression results from not being able to see a way out of your current situation. You have too much time to dwell on past or potential problems. As with loneliness and boredom, the best way to combat depression is by staying busy. Work on improving your base camp or your wilderness skills.

CHAPTER 2

Building a GOOD Kit

When it comes time to "get out of Dodge" (GOOD) it is important to have a kit, which is what you will grab and go with when the time comes. It contains everything you need to live for the first few days of your evasion.

When putting together a kit, base it on the "rule of threes." The rule of threes says that you can live about 3 seconds without thinking, 3 minutes without air, 3 hours without shelter, 3 days without water, and 3 weeks without food. Beyond these times, you will begin to suffer adverse affects, and if they continue long enough you will die.

Although most things in the GOOD kit are physical items, a portion of what is discussed here involves the planning that went into assembling the kit in the first place.

To help you think, include a copy of your evasion intelligence plan in the kit. This is the thinking you've done about your planned evasion over time. You may want to include a survival reference book (perhaps this one) and, if you have religious tendencies, a Bible or prayer book.

Air is generally not a problem in a wilderness area. In fact, it is probably fresher and cleaner than that of any city you just left. Just be sure that you do not do anything to restrict your access to fresh air, such as building a fire in a closed space, which uses up all your oxygen.

Shelter is important for the wilderness evader. In a harsh environment you must have shelter. You need to get out of the wind and the rain, protect yourself from the sun, and maintain your body temperature.

A fresh supply of water is essential. Your GOOD kit should contain an initial supply of water. However, water is heavy, and you will not be able to carry more than 1 or 2 days' supply of water. Thereafter, you will have to obtain water from such natural sources as streams, lakes, and springs. You should carry a portable water filter and water purification chemicals (such as iodine). Because water is effectively purified by boiling, you should also have a container in which to boil water. This can be your mess kit or something as simple as a tin can. Once water is collected and purified, it needs to be stored. For this you need some type of storage container. I recommend water bladders, such as the CamelBak hydration system or similar collapsible containers.

Finally, add food and methods of food procurement to your kit. Food may be commercial freeze-dried foods, military MREs, or various mixtures like trail-mix and bannock. Items for procuring food should include a field guide of edible wild plants in your area, a fishing kit, and various traps (such as the 110 Conibear).

BUILDING A GOOD KIT

EQUIPMENT LIST

Category	Equipment
WATER	Canteens, water bladder, water filter, water purification means (e.g., iodine crystals)
SHELTER	Clothing for outdoor activity, sleeping bag and ground pad, tent, or tarp
FIRE	Matches in waterproof case, magnesium fire starter, tinder
FOOD	MREs, dried foodstuffs, fishing kit, traps, snare wire, and other items to procure game
FIRST AID AND HYGIENE	Personal toiletries, first aid kit, herbal remedies
COMMUNICATIONS	Family Radio Service and General Mobile Radio Service, general-coverage AM/FW/shortwave, radio, ham radio, batteries and a way to recharge them (e.g., solar panel)
LIGHTS	Flashlights, light-emitting diode (LED) lights, lanterns, chemical lights, candles
TOOLS	Large knife, multi-tool, hatchet, sharpening stone, .22-caliber "survival rifle," repair kit (e.g., wire, superglue, duct tape, nails, cord, awl, thread), tools (e.g., pliers, hammer, saw, hand drill)

Too often people think of survival in terms of having only minimal equipment. This is often the case, but usually not as a matter of choice. When assembling your GOOD kit think in terms of an extended camping trip, not a survival exercise. Of course, you can only carry so much, so you'll have to prioritize. Don't overlook items that will make your life easier just because they're not "survival" items.

Chapter 3

Caches

As we saw when putting together a GOOD kit, there's a lot of gear a wilderness evader might want. But the more gear, the heavier the kit is and the more difficult to carry. This is where caches come into play. A cache is a hidden supply of food and equipment used to supplement whatever equipment is carried during the initial evasion.

Defining caching, U.S. Army Special Forces says this:

> Caching is the process of hiding equipment or materials in a secure storage place with the view to future recovery for operational use. The ultimate success of caching may well depend upon attention to detail—that is, professional competence that may seem of minor importance to the untrained eye.

Security factors, such as cover for the caching party, sterility of the items cached, and removal of even the slightest trace of the caching operations, are vital. Highly important, too, are the technical factors that govern the preservation of the items in usable condition and the recording of data essential for recovery. Successful caching entails careful adherence to the basic principles of clandestine operations, as well as familiarity with the technicalities of caching.

PLANNING A CACHE

Planning a cache involves selecting items and finding an appropriate location in which to cache them. This selection is usually not a problem as long as you take time to consider your potential needs when using the items. A cache may serve to meet emergency needs or to supplement your long-term survival requirements when you are not in a position to receive supplies from outside sources. When selecting the location for a cache site, be sure that it is suitable not only for emplacement of the cache but for recovery of items as needed.

When planning a cache, first look at the contents and intended purpose of the cache. A cache meant for emergency needs (containing, perhaps, a change of clothing, food, water, and first-aid supplies) is much different from a site consisting of several 5-gallon cans of grain to support long-term food needs. The small emergency cache may be quickly established and recovered. A cache containing large and/or numerous items requires that you are able to work in the area unobserved for fairly long time. Other items, such as medical supplies, may have a limited shelf life and require rotation to ensure effectiveness.

Cache planning also requires an ability to foresee potential future restrictions on access to your cache site. A site at the end of a lonely country road may seem an ideal location when you establish the cache, but if a year later someone builds a new house over your cache site, it becomes inaccessible. When planning a cache, be sure to consider possible future obstructions to the site. Bad luck cannot be anticipated, but it can usually be mitigated by carefully considering site location and observing the patterns of the local population.

Initial planning for a cache site may be done with a map survey. Your evasion intelligence plan contains topographic maps of your evasion area, and you can use the maps along with other information about the area to determine likely cache locations. A careful review of your maps allows you to locate areas that may be suitable for caches and to rule out those that are unsuitable because they are too close to houses, businesses, busy thoroughfares, or areas the may restrict access in the future. A good topographic map shows roads, trails, and potential concealment areas, such as wooded areas. A map survey is also essential for locating landmarks (e.g., road intersections, stream convergence points, waterfalls) to use as reference points when locating the cache site for recovery.

The map survey will give you several potential cache sites, but personal observation of the selected areas is essential to making a final site selection. When visiting potential cache sites you should have your maps with you, along with a compass, measuring device, and perhaps a global positioning system (GPS) device to record exact locations and your observations at the site. It is important, as well, to carry a probe or small folding shovel to determine soil content and ease of digging if you are planning a buried cache.

When selecting a cache site, you must ensure your being able to locate and recover the cache after several months or, perhaps, years. A cache site may seem ideal in every regard, but if there are not specific landmarks that can be used to locate it in the future, the site is no good. It is also important to consider changing seasons and weather conditions with regard to site location. Will changes in foliage leave the cache site dangerously exposed or inaccessible? Will snow and frozen ground make retrieval of items impossible during the winter months?

Once you have found a suitable location for your cache, you must prepare simple and unmistakable instructions for locating its site. You must not rely on your memory. The instructions should be clear enough so that someone who has never been in the area could use them to recover the cache. The instructions should begin with a general area description noting the nearest town, village, or major identifiable area. Next comes an intermediate reference point, a durable location in the general area. This can be the only bridge on a given road, a road intersection, a cemetery entrance, or another site sure not to be changed during the life of your cache. Last you designate a final reference point that meets the following criteria:

- Can be located by following simple instructions from the intermediate reference point
- Will remain fixed throughout the life of your cache
- Must be near enough to the cache to locate the cache by precise measurements from the final reference point

It may be possible to use the same object as both the intermediate reference point and the final reference point as long as this does not result in any confusion regarding the location of the cache.

To pinpoint the exact location of the cache you describe a specific measurement along a defined line from the final reference point. For example: "The cache is 20 feet from center pillar on the west side of the bridge. Measure from the base of the pillar along a magnetic azimuth of 255 degrees. The cache is buried approximately 1 foot below the surface of the ground at the base of the boulder."

The cache may also be located directly beside the final reference point if this provides for a suitable cache location. For example: "The cache is buried approximately 1 foot below the surface of the ground on the inside of the center pillar on the west side of the bridge."

METHODS OF CACHING

Next come methods of caching. For the purposes of this book caching methods are divided into burial, submersion, and concealment.

Burial

Burial is generally the best method for maintaining long-term security of your caches. However, there are certain disadvantages to buried caches. First, burial almost always requires extensive packaging of the cached material. Second, establishing and recovering a buried cache require tools (at least something with which to dig) and are generally time consuming. Finally, a buried cache can be difficult to locate. Even with these disadvantages, however, burial is the most common method of caching.

When you are burying cache, it is important to consider drainage of the ground in which the cache is to be placed. Moisture is one of the greatest enemies to cached items, so it is essential that a cache be placed where standing water will not become a problem. If your cache site is near a stream or river, make sure that it is dug above the high-water line and above possible flood lines so that it will not be uncovered by water flow.

The natural vegetation around the cache site is also an important consideration. The root system of deciduous tress can make digging difficult, though coniferous trees have a less extensive system of roots. Coniferous trees also tend to grow in fairly well-drained soil.

Finally, consider ground cover. Grasses may be difficult to remove and replace while establishing a cache, while humus is much easier to remove and replace in a manner that will not disclose the location of the cache. If the cache must be buried or recovered in winter, it is important to take into account snow depth and the possibility that frozen ground may make digging extremely difficult or impossible.

Submersion

Submersion consists of establishing a cache below the surface of the water. Submersion has the same packaging requirements as burial, but to an even greater degree you must be absolutely sure the package is waterproof. Establishing a submerged cache requires that the person doing the caching be able to dive (or at least have a strong swimming capability) to ensure that the cache is properly anchored. Because they are so hard to establish and recover, submerged caches are best used only on rare occasions when burial or concealment is not an option and when dealing specifically with maritime-trained personnel. As with a buried cache, it is important to consider weather effects on the cache. A submerged cache may become totally inaccessible if the water in which the cache is submerged is frozen.

Concealment

Concealment makes use of natural or man-made features to hide the cache. It requires less effort and equipment than burial or submersion. As an example, a concealment cache may be hidden in an abandoned building, in a dry cave, under a culvert, underneath ruins, or beneath a natural deadfall. The primary disadvantage to concealment is the possibility of accidental discovery. Therefore, concealment is best used in remote areas or when rapid access to the cached materials is required.

PACKAGING

Proper packaging of cached material is essential to ensuring that the material is serviceable when recovered.

The method of packaging is determined by the number, size, shape, and weight of the items to be cached. Another consideration when deciding on packaging is the method of recovery of the cached items. A cache designed to be recovered by one person and moved from the area should be limited to no more than 45 pounds total recoverable weight. If a cache contains emergency survival items (e.g., food, water, first-aid supplies) it is important to remember to provide a method for them to be carried from the site. Thirty pounds of loose equipment may be impossible for one person to carry, and trying to carry such items in the cache container may prove no more effective. However, a small rucksack included in the cache allows these items to be quickly loaded and easily carried away.

When you package items it is important to consider all the factors that may affect the cache, such as moisture, temperatures, pressure, insects and bacteria in the soil, and any animals that may be attracted to the cache. With this in mind, take the following steps to package material properly:

- Inspecting cached material—Ensure that all items to be cached are functional, complete, and free of

CACHES

corrosive substances. It is of no benefit to cache a radio that has no antenna or to cache batteries leaking their acid.
- Cleaning—Next all items to go in the cache must be cleaned. All dirt, mildew, mold, rust and the like must be removed from items before they are cached.
- Drying—It is most important that items placed into cache are free of moisture. For items that are not particularly affected by heat, you can dry them in an oven at 110 degrees Fahrenheit for one hour.
- Coating with protective material—All metal parts (e.g., weapons, tools, parts) should be coated with oil to prevent rust.
- Wrapping—Items should be wrapped to protect them from the elements. Ideal wrapping material is waterproof, flexible enough to fit closely around the items, and tough enough so that it will not tear during the caching process. Some possibilities are heavy-duty aluminum foil, wax paper, or commercial shrink wrap. It is important to make sure that all seams of the wrapping material are sealed. (I generally use an inner wrapping of aluminum foil and an outer wrapping of waxed paper. This can be done by completely taping all seams and then coating the package with paraffin wax. Simply dip the entire package into hot paraffin or by brush melted paraffin onto the outside of the package.) Items should be wrapped separately so that a leak in one package does not destroy everything in the cache. If there is any technical or specialized equipment in the cache, be sure to include instructions for using it.
- Packing in the outer container—Once the items to be cached are wrapped they are packed into the outer container. Ideally, the outer container should be waterproof and airtight when sealed, resistant to insects and bacteria, lightweight, noiseless when handled (e.g., no rattling handles or rustling

plastic), and capable of withstanding the pressure of burial or submersion. Some common items for outer containers are PVC pipe, military ammunition cans, and 5-gallon plastic buckets with airtight seals. Items should be packed in the outer container so that they don't shift, and all items should be padded to withstand rough handling. Before sealing the outer container, add a long-lasting desiccant to absorb any remaining moisture once it is sealed.

After sealing the outer container, test for leaks by submerging it in water and watching for bubbles. If possible, use hot water for this test because it will reveal leaks that may not be detected by cold-water submersion.

Once the cache has been properly packed, it can be transported to the site and hidden. If it is to be buried, dig a hole deep enough to cover the outer container plus a minimum of 12 inches. At least a foot of covering soil is necessary to ensure that the cache isn't exposed by soil erosion or the activity of people passing through the area. When establishing the cache, you'll probably find that it takes longer than you first expected to make the site undetectable. You should plan for a couple hours on site to properly establish a cache of all but the smallest size. Furthermore, unless the cache site is in a very remote location, much of your work will have to be done at night to avoid casual observation and chance passersby.

THE CACHE REPORT

The final step in establishing your cache is to prepare a written cache report. The report should include the following:

- Type of cache (buried, submerged, concealed)
- A complete inventory of all items in the cache
- General area description

- Intermediate reference point description
- Final reference point and exact cache location (include measurements from the final reference point, GPS coordinates, burial depths, and other relevant facts)
- Sketches and diagrams
- Emplacement details
- Dates of emplacement and expiration dates of any perishable items
- Recovery instructions and special details not covered elsewhere in the report

Your reports must be kept secret—you don't want to compromise the cache (and perhaps any associated evasion plan). Cache reports may be included with your evasion intelligence plan or stored in a separate location from which they can be recovered during the initial stages of evasion.

CHAPTER 4

Getting There

OK, you've put together a GOOD kit and maybe established a cache or two. You've thought about the possibility of having to drop out of sight in the backwoods for a while, and you've made the decision that the time to go is now. Just how do you get there?

First, let's assume that you are not grabbing your kit and diving out your bedroom window at 2:00 A.M. as some of the alphabet soup boys make a warrantless forced entry at the front door. If that's the case, just pray that your luck holds long enough for you to get out of range and you don't end up like Sammy Weaver (Randy Weaver's son who was slain by federal agents in Ruby Ridge, Idaho), shot in the back as you run for safety.

In this case, let's say you realize that you need to drop out of sight for a while, but you're not necessarily on the run. Begin by closing up your house as if you were going on vacation. You may want to send letters to your telephone and utility services instructing them to suspend service on a given date (not, however, on the date you're to depart).

Plan on leaving your vehicle at home or perhaps moving it to a long-term storage area. Do not plan on taking it with you.

While making your departure preparations, avoid drawing any particular attention to your activities. Keep things at a low key and don't even hint at what you have in mind. If anyone asks, you are planning a vacation or perhaps a business trip. In fact, it's ideal if you can depart on a real vacation or business trip and disappear from there.

Do not burn any bridges behind you. It may be that you'll return to your home and your life in a few weeks or months. Maybe not, but don't lock yourself out of that possibility by doing something stupid.

You should have already planned how you will get to your evasion area. Travel by air is not really an option: the "air nazis" with their ID checks, paper trails, and personal searches keep you from any freedom to travel in private. Travel by bus or train can be an option. Renting a vehicle that gets dropped off at a distant destination is also a choice. This is common with moving vans and raises no particular flags. Such vehicles are sometimes overlooked by investigators trying to track you. If you can rent it in a name other than your own, so much the better.

Don't travel directly to your planned evasion area. Rent a vehicle and drive in one direction. Drop the rental off at a distant destination and take a train for the next leg of your journey. Hike to a new area and take a bus to the next destination. Your initial direction of travel in a rental vehicle (which may be traced back to you) can serve as misdirection. On the other hand, your circumstances may allow you to simply pick up your gear and hike into the mountains on Friday afternoon and be long gone before anyone misses you on Monday morning.

It is essential that you plan your initial movement to leave as few traces as possible and for whatever you must leave to be of no value to anyone trying to follow you or to lead to a dead end.

GETTING THERE

Think carefully about anything during your initial movement that may leave a clue to your destination or direction of travel. Make absolutely sure that the final leg of movement to your evasion area leaves no clues for anyone to follow.

Once you've made it to your planned evasion area and your base camp, it is time to settle down and stay out of sight. You've made it into the first stage of your evasion, and you are probably OK, with little close or active pursuit. However, this is not the time to get complacent. Make sure that you're doing everything you can to keep a low profile.

If searchers or investigators find no trace of you in the first couple of weeks, they commonly put your case on the shelf for a month or so. Most people do not escape into the wilderness. The investigator is giving you time to settle into your new life and leave a clue he can follow. A phone call, credit card purchase, withdrawal at an ATM can all be quickly traced and pinpoint your exact location. Be especially careful 6 to 8 weeks after your disappearance because investigators will be taking a second, closer look at records for some clue to your location. There may come a time when you need to make contact with the outside world, e.g., for resupply of things you used during your initial weeks of hiding out, but take a moment to ensure that this contact does not leave a traceable clue and give away your location.

Chapter 5

Resupply Systems

We've looked at caches as a means of having supplies available at a predetermined location, however it may not always be possible or desirable to establish caches in a given area.

There are two basic ways of getting resupplied. The first is to have someone you trust send items to you; the second is to purchase items through a retailer and have them shipped to you. In each case, however, you must have a destination to which items can be shipped.

For items that can be sent via U.S. mail you can have these items sent to general delivery to any U.S. post office. General delivery does not require that you establish a post office box or other type of account with the post office. There is no fee to use general delivery (other than postage required to mail the package in the first place), and while you will likely be asked to present identification to pick up your general delivery mail, as long as the names on your ID and on your package match you simply pick up your package and go. General delivery is defined in postal regulations as follows:

D930 General Delivery and Firm Holdout Summary
D930 describes the intent of general delivery . . .
1.0 General Delivery
1.1 Purpose
General delivery is intended primarily as a temporary means of delivery:
    a. For transients and customers not permanently located.
    b. For customers who want post office box service when boxes are unavailable.
1.2 Service Restrictions
General delivery is available at only one facility under the administration of a multifacility post office. A postmaster may refuse or restrict general delivery:
    a. To a customer who is unable to present suitable identification.
    b. To a customer whose mail volume or service level (e.g., mail accumulation) cannot reasonably be accommodated.
1.3 Delivery to Addressee
A general delivery customer can be required to present suitable identification before mail is given to the customer.
1.4 Holding Mail
General delivery mail is held for no more than 30 days, unless a shorter period is requested by the sender. Subject to 1.2 general delivery mail may be held for longer periods if requested by the sender or addressee.

Items may also be sent by commercial parcel shippers (e.g., United Parcel Service, Federal Express), but these shippers must have a specific street address where they can deliver the package, not a post office box. By law these commercial shippers may not deliver to a U.S. post office, but private mail companies (e.g., Mail

Boxes Etc.) can and do receive packages from commercial shippers. Many private mail companies allow you to do a one-time drop shipment to their location for a small service fee. When traveling, I have had UPS packages delivered to a Mail Boxes Etc. location for a service fee of $3.50 per box. Because using commercial shippers and mail companies is a contractual relationship between you and these companies you can pretty much arrange whatever type of delivery, receipt, and holding requirements you are willing to pay for.

Whether you plan on using U.S. Postal Service general delivery or having a package sent to some private mail company, you must make arrangements in advance.

Of course, using this type of resupply requires that you enter a town where there is a post office or commercial mail company. The desirability of going to a town to receive a package must be weighed against the possibility of compromising your own location. However, if you are not one of the nation's "10 most wanted" this method of receiving a resupply package has limited risk. Once you have mailed your resupply package it disappears into the millions of other pieces of mail in the system. A post office receiving your general delivery package will hold it up to 30 days (maybe more if you have made arrangements), and all you need to do is pick it for up during that time. There is no effective way for anyone to determine where your package was sent once it is in the postal system, and unless you attract undue attention when you pick it up, no one will ever remember you were there.

CHAPTER 6

In and Around Town

Since we are looking at the possibility of being in and around towns, I think it is important to take a minute to consider the risks involved with coming into towns, and methods of minimizing these risks.

First, assess the risks of entering a town at all. If you are on the FBI's most-wanted list or just had a starring role on *America's Most Wanted* television show, you should avoid any town or any contact with anyone other than your most trusted friends. Barring these extremes, however, it is probably safe to enter towns on an infrequent basis.

When you do go into a town it is important to blend in with the population. If you are dirty and look like you have been living in the backwoods for the past month you will be remembered. You will also be remembered if you are clean but dressed like "Buckskin Bob." However, if you are dressed in jeans, a shirt, and boots you will pass for just another working stiff.

Have a plan when you enter a town. Why are you going into town? If you plan to pick up a general delivery mail package or buy something at a store, do so and then leave town. Do not loiter anywhere or come into unnecessary contact with other people. Simply do what you have to and move on. When you prepared your evasion intelligence package, you should have obtained information about the location of the post office, store, or any other facility you might want to use. Before going into town consult your maps; know where you're going and the quickest way out of town when you're done.

Although it may not be totally out of place to see someone with a backpack, most people don't wander around town with them, so conceal yours outside the town and recover it on the way out. If you know you'll be picking up supplies and need a way to carry them, the backpack may be a necessity, but know that it makes you different from 99 percent of others on the street.

Here are things to consider when entering a town:

- Be clean and presentable. Don't stand out from the crowd.
- Don't loiter. Police tend to notice strangers just hanging around with no apparent purpose. A local busybody also tends to report these "suspicious persons" to the police.
- Don't visit the same stores, facilities, or services frequently or regularly. If you have been to any of these within a couple of months, don't go there again for some time. Avoid being remembered.
- Don't hang around town at night (after normal business hours). Don't wander through purely residential areas. You will likely be noticed, if not actually stopped and asked to explain yourself.
- Plan any trip to a town to keep it as short and low-key as possible. Get in, accomplish your business, and leave quickly—and with no one remembering that you were there.

CHAPTER 7

Evading Pursuit

OK, you're off, heading into the mountains with the opposition in hot pursuit. You have a couple hours' lead or maybe only several minutes. Speed is useful to initially put distance between yourself and your pursuers, but you should never sacrifice caution in favor of speed. Unless your pursuers can actually see you, they don't know exactly where you are. They may have a general idea, maybe even a fairly accurate idea, but the advantage remains yours.

As soon as you get into terrain offering any type of concealment, slow down and think. Use the terrain to your advantage to mask your movement and cover your back trail. Stealth is the way to evade pursuit. If you move steadily and cautiously, taking advantage of terrain, vegetation, and the like to stay hidden, you force your pursuers to break off pursuit and begin a search. Remember, they can't chase you if they don't know where you are.

The longer you can go without your pursuers' determining a location for you, the greater your advantage becomes. This is why stealth is so important. An uninjured man traveling over unbroken ground can maintain an average pace of 4 miles per hour. This pace is faster than a casual walk but is definitely not running. Allowing for caution in movement and for rest, this pace can be reduced by half, to 2 miles per hour. Thus from your last known location you could be 2 miles away in 1 hour. However, because you could have traveled in any direction from your last known location, your pursuers must search the area of a circle that is 4 miles in diameter. A little arithmetic lets us determine the area of the circle to be just over 12.5 square miles. In 6 hours you could have traveled 12 miles, giving us a circle diameter of 24 miles and an area of 452.39 square miles to be searched. After a full day (24 hours) without searchers being able to locate you, you could have traveled 48 miles, giving us a circle diameter of 96 miles and an area of 7,238.22 square miles to be searched.

This is all theoretical, and when you draw the circle around your last known location on a map, there will be places that you obviously could not be. For example, if a lake takes up part of the circle, the chances are pretty good that you are not hiding at the bottom of the lake. However, this formula is fairly accurate for actual searches. With each passing hour that you remain undetected, the circle continues to expand. However, if searchers are able to deter-

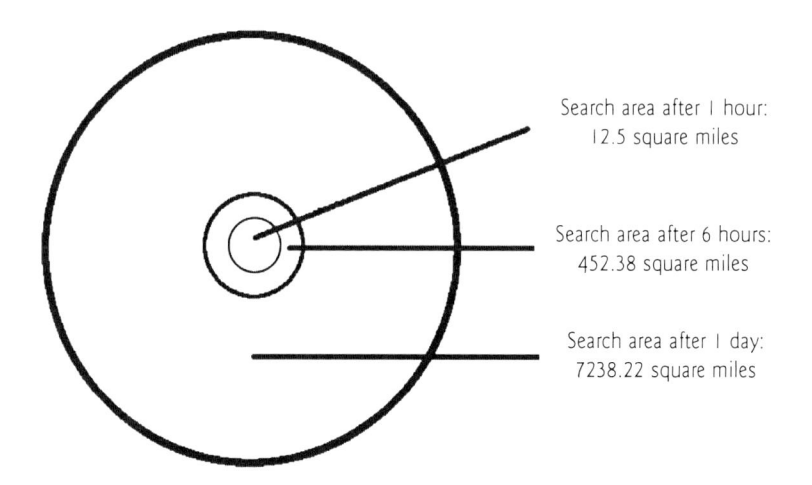

Search area after 1 hour:
12.5 square miles

Search area after 6 hours:
452.38 square miles

Search area after 1 day:
7238.22 square miles

mine a location for you because you were spotted or they found your last campsite, tracks, trash, or other sign left by you, they again have a "last known location," and the search area starts to shrink in favor of the searchers. Therefore, remember that stealth is your salvation. Take your time, leave no trace, and think!

Don't let panic take control of you. Assess your current situation. How many people are searching for you? How close are they? Are they armed? Do they have dogs? What equipment do you have with you? If you don't have your GOOD kit, what's in your pockets (pocket knife, matches, compass, cord, or wire)? Are you injured? Are you armed? Are you familiar with the area you are in? Stop and listen. Can you hear your pursuers? Do you hear them moving through the brush? Can you hear shouts, conversation, radio noise, vehicles? As you continue to evade, can you circle around on your back trail and get a look at your pursuers? Don't spend an inordinate amount of time watching them; while you are watching them they may see you. Quickly gather whatever information you can about your pursuers and work that into your evasion plan. This information will allow you to know the odds against you.

OK, so who's on your trail? Is a military squad, well trained and well armed, pursuing you? Are your pursuers a couple of guys who were guarding a marijuana field you stumbled across? If you know that you can slip away from your pursuers, now is the time to do it. Stay concealed, stick to cover, and get out of the area. This early in the game your pursuers probably aren't trackers, so unless you are leaving more signs behind you than a Mardi Gras parade, you should be able to just disappear. Now if your pursuers want you, they must bring in trackers to pick up your trail and resume the chase.

TRACKING AND COUNTERTRACKING

A really good tracker can follow you where the average man will detect no evidence of your passing. However, there are damn few really good trackers.

Whenever you move through an area, you leave some sign of our passing, no matter how faint that sign may actually be. By taking care to avoid leaving a major sign, and by employing various techniques to slow and defeat the tracker, it is usually possible to make a successful evasion.

When a tracker follows someone he tries to build a mental picture of the person he is tracking. Is this person healthy? What is his state of physical fitness? Is he injured? How is this person equipped, and how well trained is he? What is his state of mind? Does he know he is being followed? To answer these questions, the tracker will look for signs and indicators left by the person he is following. For example, a tracker finding the camp where the evader spent the night can determine that the fugitive has a means to light a fire and maybe has an ax or large knife to split wood. He may also be able to determine that the evader is carrying food from any leftovers or discarded wrappings.

SIGNS TRACKERS LOOK FOR

The signs and indicators sought by a tracker can be divided into five major categories: displacement, stains, trash, activities, and weather effects.

Displacement

Displacement is when an object has been moved from its original location by some action of the evader. This includes such things as soil displaced as the evader walks up a hill or a footprint in the mud beside a stream.

Stains

Stains are the discoloration of areas on the trail the tracker is following. Mud tracked onto rocks as the evader crosses a stream is an example. If the evader is injured, blood may stain the ground and surrounding vegetation as the evader moves through the area.

Trash

Trash is exactly what one would expect: items brought into an area and discarded by the evader. Empty food packaging is an example of trash that the tracker can use to build a profile of the evader.

Activities

Activities are those things done by the evader that help the tracker build a mental picture of the person he is following. For example, if a tracker determines that the evader is walking backward or doing other things to attempt to confuse his pursuers, that clearly indicates that the evader suspects he is being followed.

Weather Effects

The effect the weather has had on the various signs the tracker is following also serve to provide him with information about the evader. A tracker can tell the approximate age of a footprint by the way the weather has aged it. A rusted tin can was obviously discarded quite some time ago, but a can with a clean, sharp edge where it has been opened was discarded recently.

MINIMIZING SIGNS OF YOUR PRESENCE

Keeping in mind that the tracker must have some type of sign or indicator to keep him on your trail. Let's look at ways to reduce the signs and remove the indicators.

Trash

First and foremost the evader should simply be careful not to leave obvious sign along the trail. Don't discard anything where it may be discovered by a tracker.

Footprints

Wearing soft-soled footgear (such as moccasins) avoids the sharp outline left by hard-soled boots and limits displacement of soil as you walk. Some have suggested wearing a covering over the boots to disguise the tracks. This does conceal the sole pattern of your boots but will not completely disguise your trail.

In an area with established trails, an evader moving along one of the trails can blend his tracks with those of others who've passed that way and have his tracks covered by those who pass along the trail after him. If the evader can walk along a paved road, he removes all tracks but takes the chance of being observed by others using the road.

When a tracker follows your footprints, he notes the sole pattern of your boots and any irregularities in the tread. An effective way to confuse a tracker or throw him off your trail is to change your boots to a pair with a different sole pattern or to soft-soled footgear that leaves no distinctive pattern. By moving onto a well-used trail or paved road and then changing footgear prior to leaving the trail, you make it extremely difficult for a tracker to pick up your trail again.

Time and Weather

If you are in excellent physical shape and used to traveling across rough terrain, it is possible to completely outdistance a pursuer. Understanding that weather serves to fade tracks and wipe out signs, rapid movement in a heavy rain or snowstorm gives you distance and wipes out your tracks. It is important to remember, however, that although speed is useful, it should be used as a specific technique. Relying on speed alone means that you are failing to employ more effective techniques. Rapid movement leaves more sign than slow careful movement, and a tracker may be able to guess your destination and position interceptors ahead of you.

ACTIVE ANTITRACKING TECHNIQUES

These techniques reduce the sign you leave along the trail and may serve to slow or confuse a tracker. These techniques also do not specifically reveal to the tracker that you know you are being followed. However, it may become necessary to take additional steps to lose a pursing tracker. Active antitracking techniques let the tracker know that you are aware that you're being followed but also may make the tracker completely lose your trail.

The Screened Turn

A useful technique to hide your trail is the 90-degree screened turn. As your trail takes you past a large tree (about 14 inches or more in diameter) continue past the tree about 10 or

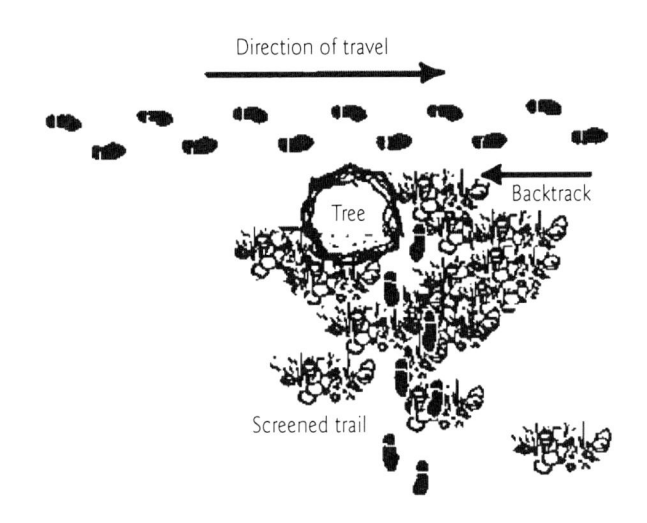

12 paces. Then back up to the forward side of the tree, very carefully stepping in your own tracks. At the forward side of the tree make a 90-degree turn. The tree serves to screen your turn from the pursuing tracker.

The reason this technique works is that a tracker follows your trail looking for sign that indicates your direction of travel. He does not see every footprint that you leave. The tracker seeing sign indicating that you moved in a particular direction will continue to search for sign along your general direction of movement. This usually causes him to pass the area where you changed direction if it is screened from his view.

In time, once the tracker realizes that he's lost your trail, he'll return to the last sign he had of you and will begin a search for sign to pick up your trail. He will very likely find the new trail you made after making the turn, but it has cost him time, and you have gained a greater lead.

Cut the Corner

As you approach a road make a 45- to 60-degree turn to the left or right. When you reach the road, move along it in the direc-

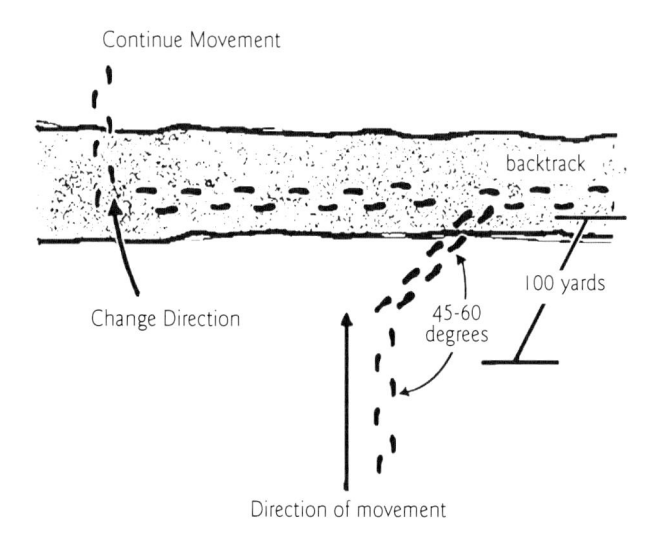

```
                Continue Movement
                      ↑
    ═══════════════════════════════════════
                                 backtrack
    ─ ─ ─ ─ ─ ─ ─ ─ ─ ─ ─ ─ ─ ─ ─ ─ ─ ─
    ═══════════════════════════════════════
                              ↖  100 yards
         Change Direction   45-60
                            degrees
                              ↑
                              ↑
                   Direction of movement
```

tion of your turn, perhaps leaving some sign along the edge of the road. After a short distance reverse your direction and move beyond the point where you originally entered the road. Be careful to leave no sign as you move back down the road. When you have moved a sufficient distance down the road, leave it and continue in your original direction of travel.

This technique serves to make a tracker believe that you've traveled along a road in one direction when you have actually crossed the road and continued your original direction of travel. Once a tracker determines that you did not go along the road (or if he suspects that you have used this technique) he'll search for sign of your crossing along the far side of the road. Because you can move rapidly along the road without leaving sign, I recommend that you backtrack at least several hundred yards before crossing the road. This increases the distance the tracker must search to find your trail and may cause him to miss it entirely.

The Slip-Stream

This technique is very similar to the cut-the-corner technique described above. When approaching a known stream, make a turn

EVADING PURSUIT 45

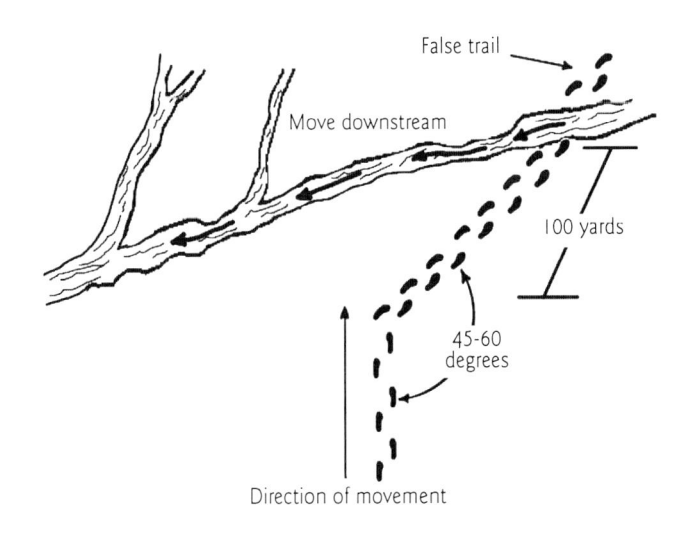

Figure: False trail technique showing movement downstream along a stream, with a false trail exit at 45-60 degrees, continuing 100 yards in the original direction of movement.

of 45 to 60 degrees toward upstream. Enter the stream, move upstream a short distance, lay a false trail (e.g., footprints in the dirt, mud on a rock), and exit on the far side. Carefully reenter the stream and proceed downstream. This technique may conceal your tracks while in the stream (depending on the composition of the stream bed), but remember that floating debris and silt may indicate your presence to people downstream and that you will have to exit the stream sometime.

Unexpected Direction Changes

Another effective method of causing a tracker to lose your trail is to change direction at an extreme angle of 120 to 160 degrees. This does not take you directly back the way you came (as a 180-degree turn would), and this type of a turn is unexpected to the tracker pursuing you.

When you do the direction change on hard or rocky soil it is difficult for the tracker to detect; he'll usually overshoot the end of your tracks and go on, looking for sign in your original direction of travel. Eventually the tracker will realize that you must have turned off your original direction of travel, and he will return to the last sign he had of you and begin to search for your new trail.

Take care not to make a turn greater than 160 degrees: the trackers may discover signs of your coming back on your own trail, or you may actually run into trackers who are closer than you believed them to be. Extreme direction changes may work more than once, but once a tracker has discovered your technique he will quickly look for unexpected turns after he loses your tracks rather than continuing to search in your original direction of travel. Still, having to conduct a search to pick up your new trail after each major direction change costs the tracker time and gains lead time for you.

ANTITRACKING MYTHS

There are a few myths about antitracking that should be looked at to keep you from wasting your time.

Walking Backward

First, consider walking backward to leave a set of tracks pointing in the opposite direction of your route. This is one technique most commonly suggested by people who have no clue about tracking. Any tracker who is not a complete idiot will immediately see this techniques for what it is. A person walking backward takes smaller, less sure steps. The impact marks of the tracks are reversed. When you walk forward, your heel strikes the ground first and you roll forward onto the ball of your foot. When you walk backward, the ball of your foot strikes the ground first and you roll back onto your heel. Walking backward lets the tracker know that you suspect you are being followed and are taking steps to fool him, so he will be more alert to antitracking techniques. Furthermore, walking backward slows you down, causing you to lose valuable lead time. Don't waste your time with backward walking—it doesn't work!

Faked Animal Tracks

People who should know better sometimes suggest leaving imitation animal tracks by attaching carved hooves to the bottom of boots. This may serve to briefly confuse an inexperienced tracker, anyone who has actually followed the tracks of real animals will immediately notice that the tracks left by carved hooves has something missing: two additional legs. I haven't seen too many elk walking around on two legs, and the only moose that walks on two legs is Bullwinkle. Furthermore, animals tend to wander, stopping to feed. An evader moves purposefully and with an intended destination, in a very unanimal-like pattern. Carrying fake animal hooves to tie onto the bottom of your boots is a waste of space and time. Simply changing your boots to a pair with a different sole pattern or changing to soft-soled moccasins is much more effective.

If the human tracker is unable to maintain your track, he may bring in a dog team to assist in the pursuit. So, next let's take a look at evading dogs.

EVADING DOGS

Being tracked by dogs is a serious problem for an evader. Let me begin by saying that it is extremely difficult to evade a dog that has your scent and wants to follow you. The tricks seen in the movies to throw off a dog simply don't work.

Tracking dogs can be divided into two major categories: air trackers and ground trackers. The air tracker picks up your scent on the wind. Any hunter knows the principle of staying downwind of an animal he is stalking. The air tracker dog is simply trained to follow a particular scent, to locate that scent in the air, and to lead his handlers to whoever is giving off the scent.

The ground tracker picks up your scent from the ground and objects near the ground that you touch as you move through an area. The ground tracker dog will follow your specific path though an area, while the air tracker dog will seek its own path, working downwind from you, as it follows your scent on the wind. Dogs have a sense of smell that is thousands of times greater than that of humans.

Tracking dogs do not track you alone, however. They are accompanied by a dog handler and likely by other human trackers or searchers. An experienced dog handler with well-trained dogs can be very difficult to elude, especially when the dog handler is a tracker in his own right. The dog follows the scent while the handler/tracker looks for visible sign. If the dog loses the scent in some area, the human tracker may be able to pick up the trail from visible sign.

Dogs do have certain weaknesses that can be exploited by an evader. Dogs track best in cool, moist environments. In hot, dry, windy areas dogs tire quickly and often lose the scent they are following. Tracker dogs are pretty much restricted to working with one handler. Furthermore, tracker dogs are expensive to train and maintain, so they may not be generally available.

There are two major aspects to evading tracker dogs. As said previously, it is very difficult to evade a dog that has your scent and wants to follow you. So, first, you must make the dog lose your scent, and, second, you must make the dog not want to follow you. Because tracker dogs work with a single handler, you must break down the trust between the handler and the dog and make the handler not want to follow you.

Techniques for Evading Tracker Dogs

- Cross obstacles that are difficult or impossible for the dog to follow. An evader may be able to scramble up a cliff (or rappel down) where a dog can't follow.
- Make several erratic direction changes. This does not particularly confuse the dog but may cause the handler to believe the dog has lost the scent.
- If evading air tracker dogs, move with the wind. This causes the scent to be blowing away from the tracker dogs, making it much harder to follow.
- Mix your scent with that of other humans. This may confuse the dog and slow it down.
- Snares, punji stakes, or several fishhooks spaced along a strong line woven through the brush along your back trail will often entangle or injure pursuing dogs. When the dogs are injured, they lose their interest in the pursuit.
- Set traps to stop the dog handler. Remember that a specific handler controls the tracker dogs. If the

EVADING PURSUIT

handler cannot continue the pursuit the dogs will have to stop with him. Even if the dogs are working free (not on a lead), if the handler is disabled the dog will have to be called back.

Myths About Evading Dogs

- Hiding under water and breathing through a reed or tube. The best you can hope for is that the dogs will simply track you to the water's edge and become confused. However, dog handlers and other trackers accompany dogs. You have to be deep enough so that you can't be seen by the handlers (or by the dog itself). But if you are this deep you won't be able to breathe through a tube for very long. Furthermore, dogs have been known to locate bodies that are underwater.
- Sprinkling pepper or other irritant on the ground to "burn out" the dog's nose as it follows your scent. This has no effect on an air tracker dog and almost no effect on a ground tracker. The dog will detect pepper and other like scents long before it has the opportunity to snort any up its nose. In fact, if the dog does snort a little pepper it will likely just make the dog sneeze, thereby cleaning out its nose and letting it follow your scent more easily. An extremely heavy concentration of pepper on the ground might keep the dog from finding your scent directly under the pepper, but any amount of pepper you could reasonably expect to carry with you simply won't faze the dog.
- Covering yourself in manure or excrement. This does little more than make you smell like a human covered in excrement to the dog. Your human scent is still present and is not significantly masked by the odor of excrement.
- Tying plastic trash bags around your feet and legs

to avoid leaving any scent. The only really effective way to cause a dog to lose your scent is to get off the ground in a car, on a bicycle, or in a boat. You must then travel a significant distance so that the dog cannot simply reacquire your scent on the ground a few hundred yards away.

CHAPTER 8

Communications

Evasion in the wilderness does not necessarily mean that you're alone or that you'll have no contact with others. It may be important that you keep your whereabouts unknown to society at large, especially to specific portions of society, but you may have trusted friends and family you'll wish to communicate with from time to time.

TELEPHONES

In today's society, the telephone is pretty much the standard for individual communication. The telephone system is near 100-percent reliable in major industrialized countries and reasonable even in many Third World countries. However, for the telephone system to be of any use, you must have access to a telephone line (home, business, pay phone) or be near a cellular site. In remote areas neither of these options may be available. Even if you are able to find a phone in a remote area, using it could immediately pinpoint your exact location (e.g., caller ID).

Cellular Telephones

Some have suggested using cellular telephones as part of a survival communications package. Generally, "cell phones" will not be effective for your purposes.

Cell phones are basically radio transceivers. In North America, cell phones transmit in the 824-849-MHz range and receive in the 869-894-MHz range (yes, I know there are exceptions to this frequency range). Your cell phone communicates via radio with a cell site that is tied into the telephone system through a microwave link or a hardwired connection. These cell sites are located throughout the service area of your cellular company.

In urban areas these cell sites may be located every few blocks. In rural areas the cell sites are often a few miles apart. In remote areas cell sites generally don't exist. For your cellular telephone to work it must be within radio range of a cell site. Because of their operating frequency and relatively low output power, cell phones must be within a few miles of a cell site to access the site and link into the telephone system. If you currently use a cell phone, you have no doubt found that you sometimes have no signal in areas that are in no way remote. Simply put, you were not within effective radio range of a cell site (or something was blocking your transmission path). In a remote area it is highly unlikely that there will be any cell sites; therefore, there will be no signal and no communication.

RADIOS

In remote areas the best means is radio, which gives you a reliable means of communication over any distance (you can literally communicate around the world with radio). So let's take a look at radio for survival communications.

The first rule of survival communication is to have someone with whom to communicate. It does little good to carry radios for communication if there is no one prepared to receive your transmissions and reply.

Let's assume that you have planned to communicate with friends by radio. Just what type of radio do you want in a survival situation?

FRS and GMRS

The Family Radio Service (FRS) and General Mobile Radio Service (GMRS) provide great short-range communication. Although two separate services, FRS and GMRS share certain frequencies.

First let's look at the FRS. FRS radios are becoming increasingly more popular and are available in most stores that sell radios in general. FRS radios require no Federal Communications Commission (FCC) license and are designed, as the name implies, for personal (family) use in noncommercial communication. FRS radios operate with a maximum power of 500 mW (1/2 watt) on up to 14 channels. This gives an average communication range of around 2 miles, although terrain may increase or decrease this somewhat. Because of their low power and limited transmission range, FRS radios are great for use among a small group moving in a wilderness environment or working around an established base camp. The sort-range of FRS means that communications are not broadcast over half the state every time you key your radio.

The GMRS is similar to FRS and in fact shares some of the FRS frequencies. GMRS requires a FCC station license (which at the time of this writing costs $85), and the FCC will assign you a GMRS call sign. GMRS operates on 15 simplex channels, with an additional seven repeater channels. Maximum power allowed on GMRS radios is 50 watts, although hand-held GMRS radios operate on 2–5 watts. This gives you an effective communication range of up to 5 miles. GMRS is not the "business radio band" but is intended for more "formal" purposes than FRS. The licensing requirements for GMRS radios is similar to the old requirements for CB radios. When you purchase a GMRS radio, there is a license application included with the radio that you are supposed to fill out and send off to the FCC with appropriate fees. Nobody checks to make sure you sent in your application, and, unless you are interfering with licensed GMRS radio stations or using your radios for

FRS/GMRS FREQUENCIES (CHANNEL—MHz)

FRS		GMRS	
1	462.5625	1	462.5625
2	462.5875	2	462.5875
3	462.6125	3	462.6125
4	462.6375	4	462.6375
5	462.6625	5	462.6625
6	462.6875	6	462.6875
7	462.7125	7	462.7125
8	467.5625	8	462.5750
9	467.5875	9	462.6250
10	467.6125	10	462.6750
11	467.6375	11	462.5500
12	467.6625	12	462.6000
13	467.6875	13	462.6500
14	467.7125	14	462.7000
		15	462.7250

(Channels 1–7 are the same for both FRS and GMRS radios. GMRS radios operate with greater power and have greater range than FRS radios.)

some criminal purpose, I doubt the radio police will be knocking on your door anytime soon.

Both FRS and GMRS come with a continuous-tone coded squelch system (CTCSS), often advertised as "privacy codes." After choosing a operating frequency (channel), on radios with the CTCSS function you then can choose one of 38 CTCSS codes. This prevents you from hearing any transmission that does not contain the same CTCSS code. For example, if you set your radio to channel 3 and your CTCSS code to 23, you will only receive transmissions with the same 3/23 setting. Because CTCSS is sometimes billed as privacy codes, some people believe that setting a CTCSS code prevents anyone without the same code set from hearing the transmissions. This is not true. If you listen to the frequency with no CTCSS code set, you will hear all transmissions on the frequency, no matter what CTCSS code the transmitting station has set. The intent of CTCSS is to allow you to avoid receiving unwanted transmissions in an area where there are many users of the frequencies. For use in survival communications CTCSS codes are of limited value since you will probably be working in a remote area with few radio operators.

Some FRS radios have a "scramble" function that allows you to choose one of three preset codes, which prevents your transmissions from being understood by anyone not having that "scramble code" programmed. This may have some function in survival communications, but, again, unless you are operating in an area with radio operators or monitoring stations within a few miles, the value of scramble codes are questionable.

So which radio is best for short-range survival communications, FRS or GMRS? Generally, I recommend the FRS radios, unless you simply must have the additional range provided by GMRS. I keep a FRS radio in my kit at all times, even when I am carrying other radio equipment. Once you have added FRS to your personal communications package you may wonder how you managed to get along without it in the past. When choosing an FRS radio, there are a couple of points to keep in mind. First, be sure that the FRS radio you purchase operates on all 14 FRS channels (some FRS radios have only one or two channels). Also be sure that the radio you purchase operates at the full 500-mW output power (some FRS radios operate at 300 mW). Other than these points, all FRS radios made by major manufacturers are pretty much the same with regard to actual transmission and reception capability. Such additional features as ringing tones, FM broadcast-band receiver, NOAA weather band, and physical design are a matter of personal preference.

Citizens Band

Citizens band (CB) radio has been around for years, and millions of them have been sold. Most commercial truckers have CB radios in their rigs. CB radios require no FCC license and can be found just about everywhere. The fact that CB radios are everywhere means that the 40 channels assigned to the CB tend to be crowded. Many people seem to think that having a CB radio is their opportunity to act like a complete fool on the airwaves. Rather than using the radio to request or provide information or to simply have a conversation with another person, the average CB operator prattles on with a string of endless babble or floods the channel with noise, making it difficult for anyone else to actually communicate.

In addition to the drivel found on CB channels, many operators modify their radios to transmit with excessive power and outside the CB band, causing harmful interference with the ham radio 10- and 12-meter bands. So does this mean that CB has no place in survival communications?

A good-quality portable CB radio will give you a communication range of 5 or 10 miles, assuming you can get through the interference on the channel. A good-quality base station with a proper antenna will give you perhaps a 100-mile communication range (again barring heavy interference on the channel). However, as you move into more and more remote areas, interference tends to decrease along with the population.

A CB radio set up at your base camp can provide communication throughout the general area of the camp. Using directional antennas you may be able to maintain communications with someone at a significant distance from camp.

CITIZENS BAND RADIO (CB)

CB Frequencies (Channel—MHz)

1	26.965	21	27.215
2	26.975	22	27.225
3	26.985	23	27.235
4	27.005	24	27.245
5	27.015	25	27.255
6	27.025	26	27.265
7	27.035	27	27.275
8	27.055	28	27.285
9	27.065	29	27.295
10	27.075	30	27.305
11	27.085	31	27.315
12	27.105	32	27.325
13	27.115	33	27.335
14	27.125	34	27.345
15	27.135	35	27.355
16	27.155	36	27.365
17	27.165	37	27.375
18	27.175	38	27.386
19	27.185	39	27.395
20	27.205	40	27.405

Amateur (Ham) Band

Amateur band radio has the capability to provide literally around-the-world communications. For someone who needs to establish effective communication from a remote area, ham radio is definitely the way to go. Operating on the ham frequencies requires a license and assigned call sign from the FCC. A basic license requires that you pass a written exam covering operating procedures and basic electronics; for an advanced license, you must demonstrate that you are able to copy Morse code at a rate of five groups per minute. The exams are very easy; even young children hold ham radio licenses. With a few days' study you should have no problem earning your basic technician's license. At the time of this writing, exam fees are $10, and your license is good for 10 years.

If you decide to use ham radio as part of your survival communications plan, it is essential that you actually take the time to get your license. Ham radio operators take a dim view of unlicensed people messing around on the amateur band frequencies (and rightly so).

One of the many parts of the ham radio hobby is "field day" that consists of, among other things, operating radios in a field environment. There is a bunch of information available on operating radios from remote locations, allowing you to set up and run an effective ham radio station almost anywhere.

Ham radio can be run on various power output settings, thus somewhat limiting or increasing your transmission range. However, it should be clearly understood when using ham radio in a survival situation that other operators will very likely overhear your conversations. In many cases these people will come back to you just to be sociable or to make contact with someone with an out-of-area call sign. Although the FCC does not require it, most ham radio operators keep station logs in which they record their contacts and sometimes stations heard but with which they did not have contact. Understanding this, unless you are attempting to evade people with radio-direction-finding capability (and many ham radio operators have this capability), ham radio can serve as the basis for your survival communications package.

Ham radio operators have operating privileges on the following frequencies (depending on the level of license one has obtained).

AMATEUR BAND RADIO

UHF/VHF

1240 band	1240–1300 MHz
900 band	902–928 MHz
440 band	420–450 MHz
222 band	222–225 MHz
2 meters	144–148 MHz
6 meters	50.1–54 MHz

HF Bands

10 meters	28–29.7 MHz
12 meters	24.890–24.990 MHz
15 meters	21–21.450 MHz
17 meters	18.068–18.168 MHz
20 meters	14–14.450 MHz
30 meters1	0.1–10.150 MHz
40 meters	7–7.300 MHz
75/80 meters	3.5–4.0 MHz
160 meters	1.8–2.0 MHz

Morse Code

Although Morse code is not required to earn your technician-class ham radio operator's license, I believe that it is a valuable tool for the person trying to set up a communications network. It allows communication over long distances and uses low power. When conditions make communication by voice difficult or impossible, you can often still send and receive messages using Morse code. Using Morse code and a low-power radio that will literally fit in your pocket, it's possible to communicate across several states with ease.

Morse code is best mastered by learning to recognize a sound pattern as a particular letter or number, not by memorizing the dots and dashes. There are various freeware computer programs available on the Internet that you can download and use to practice Morse code. You can also purchase various cassette tapes and CDs containing Morse code study programs at places that sell ham radio equipment.

Wilderness Protocol

The wilderness protocol is used by ham radio operators operating on UHF/VHF frequencies in remote areas. The protocol asks that ham radio operators monitor the primary frequency of 146.52 MHz (and if possible the secondary frequencies of 52.525 MHz, 223.50 MHz, 446.00 MHz, and 1294.50 MHz) every 3 hours beginning at 0700 hours (7 A.M.) local time, for 5 minutes (e.g., 0700–0705, 1000–1005, 1300–1305 hours). The purpose is to allow ham radio operators in areas not covered by repeaters to have specific times for making contact for priority traffic. Although the protocol was originally developed for use by ham operators who were hiking or backpacking in the backwoods, it has become fairly common in any area without repeater coverage. I spend a fair amount of time in remote areas and make it a point to follow wilderness protocol, as do most other operators I know who spend time in the wilderness.

What does a HAM radio etiquette have to do with wilderness survival and evasion? First, anyone considering wilderness evasion ham radio. If you have your ham radio license, the wilderness protocol gives you a means of emergency communication. If you don't

MORSE CODE CHARACTER CHART

Letters

	Sound	Dot/Dash		Sound	Dot/Dash
A	didah	• –	N	dahdit	– •
B	dahdididit	– • • •	O	dahdahdah	– – –
C	dahdidahdit	– • – •	P	didahdahdit	• – – •
D	dahdidit	– • •	Q	dahdahdidah	– – • –
E	dit	•	R	didahdit	• – •
F	dididahdit	• • – •	S	dididit	• • •
G	dahdahdit	– – •	T	dah	–
H	dididit	• • • •	U	dididah	• • –
I	didit	• •	V	didididah	• • • –
J	didahdahdah	• – – –	W	didahdah	• – –
K	dahdidah	– • –	X	dahdididah	– • • –
L	didahdidit	• – • •	Y	dahdidahdah	– • – –
M	dahdah	– –	Z	dahdahdidit	– – • •

Numbers

	Sound	Dot/Dash
1	didahdahdahdah	• – – – –
2	dididahdahdah	• • – – –
3	didididahdah	• • • – –
4	dididididah	• • • • –
5	didididit	• • • • •
6	dahdidididit	– • • • •
7	dahdahdididit	– – • • •
8	dahdahdahdidit	– – – • •
9	dahdahdahdahdit	– – – – •
0	dahdahdahdahdah	– – – – –

have your ham radio license, wilderness protocol frequencies can still be programmed into a scanner, allowing you to monitor emergency traffic in your evasion area.

Scanners

A scanner is simply a receiver that listens briefly to preselected frequencies for transmissions. The scanner continues to move through these frequencies until it detects a transmission. When it finds a transmission on a selected frequency, it stops and plays the transmission. Scanners are handy for listening to police, fire department, and local service company radio transmissions to learn firsthand what's going on in the area.

Another major advantage of scanners is that they allow you to monitor several frequencies at once. You can listen for calls on a selected ham frequency, monitor communications on a local FRS net, and keep track of the local forest service without having to power up multiple radios.

General-Coverage Receivers

A general coverage receiver is the radio most of us have in our homes. It covers the AM and FM broadcast bands and possibly various shortwave frequencies. Having a small multiband, general-coverage receiver in your kit comes in handy for picking up local news and weather reports. Additionally, there is some entertainment value to being able to listen to music and talk radio shows. This entertainment helps to fight boredom and loneliness that can occur when spending weeks on end in a remote location.

NOAA Weather Band Radio

NOAA has established a system of radio transmitters throughout the United States that continuously broadcasts weather and related information. This information is updated every 1 to 3 hours and broadcast on seven frequencies between 162.40 and 162.55 MHz. Severe storm and other emergency warnings interrupt the ongoing weather broadcast, keeping you immediately informed of changing weather patterns. The weather radio transmitters broadcast in the VHF FM high-band mode, giving them an effective transmission range of about 50 miles. Most areas of the United States are covered by weather radio broadcasts, including some fairly remote areas. It pays to check to see whether you can receive weather radio broadcasts in your area and, if you can receive them, to add a radio to your kit capable of picking up these broadcasts.

The seven NWR broadcast frequencies are as follows:

>162.400 MHz
>162.425 MHz
>162.450 MHz
>162.475 MHz
>162.500 MHz
>162.525 MHz
>162.550 MHz.

Batteries

All radio equipment requires some way of powering itself. Generally, this means batteries. Some general-coverage receivers (e.g., BayGen) use a windup dynamo to produce the required electricity to run the radio. Other radios use solar panels as a source of power. All radio equipment I carry in my kit is capable of running off 1.5 V AA batteries. I also have a solar-powered battery charger that allows me to recharge batteries and keep my equipment running.

Don't underestimate the importance of having sufficient batteries (or other power sources) for your communication equipment. A radio without power is nothing but useless weight!

Antennas

The secret to transmitting and receiving with any radio is its antenna. A fair radio with a good antenna almost always gives you a better signal and clearer reception than will a great radio with a fair antenna. Unfortunately, most portable radios don't have very good antennas.

This problem is fairly easily corrected, however. Wire antennas, which are easily portable, can be built and carried with your radio equipment. Being little more than wire, resistors, and insulators, wire antennas take up little space and weight next to nothing.

When building an antenna it should be cut to match the frequency on which you plan to operate. Generally, you cut your antenna to match the half-wave of the frequency. If you plan to operate on a single frequency, you can cut the antenna to the exact half-wave length of that frequency. However, most of the time you will operate on several different frequencies within the same band. In this case, cut your antenna to a frequency in the center of the band or to match your primary frequency.

To determine the correct wire length for your half-wave antenna, divide the operating frequency in megahertz into a constant of 468. The result is the required length of wire in feet. (468 / frequency in MHz = length in feet). For example, if you are operating in the 10-meter ham radio band on 29 MHz, you need a half-wave antenna of approximately 16 feet (468 / 29 = 16.13793).

The actual wire is measured from the antenna terminal on the radio to the far end of the antenna. The end of the antenna terminates in an electrical insulator, such as a piece of PVC pipe, block of wood, or piece of plastic. The wire for the antenna can be any insulated or uninsulated copper wire strong enough to not break under its own weight. A connector for the radio's antenna terminal can be soldered to each wire antenna, or you can have a single connector with clips, allowing you to connect the wire as needed.

Vertical Antenna

The simplest antenna to make is the vertical antenna. It is just a single wire run from the radio and supported by an overhead support, such as a tree branch.

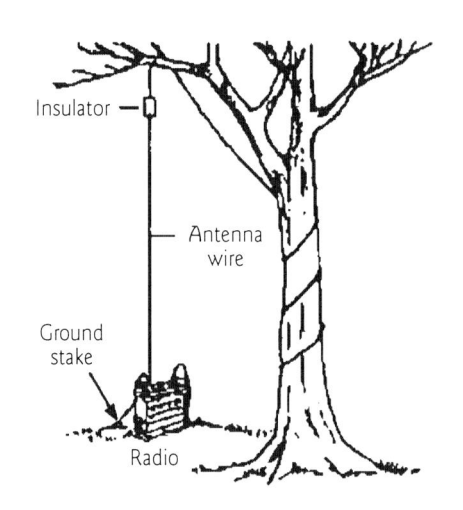

The simplest way to get your vertical antenna into a tree is to throw a rope over a branch high enough to support the antenna vertically. Connect the insulated end of your antenna to the rope and pull it into the tree. Then just use the rope to tie off the antenna and hold it in place. This vertical antenna is omni-directional, allowing you to communicate with stations you don't know the precise locations of or with mobile stations. It is definitely more efficient than the little "rubber duck" antennas that come with most portable radio equipment.

Sloping "V" Antenna

Once you have established a base camp, you may want to communicate with another station in a specific area. Communication between specific areas is best accomplished with a directional antenna. This focuses your signal in a particular direction, enhancing the receiving station's reception and limiting reception by stations for which your traffic is not intended.

The sloping V antenna works particularly well for this purpose. It is designed as a full-wavelength antenna and works even better when it is 2 or more wavelengths long.

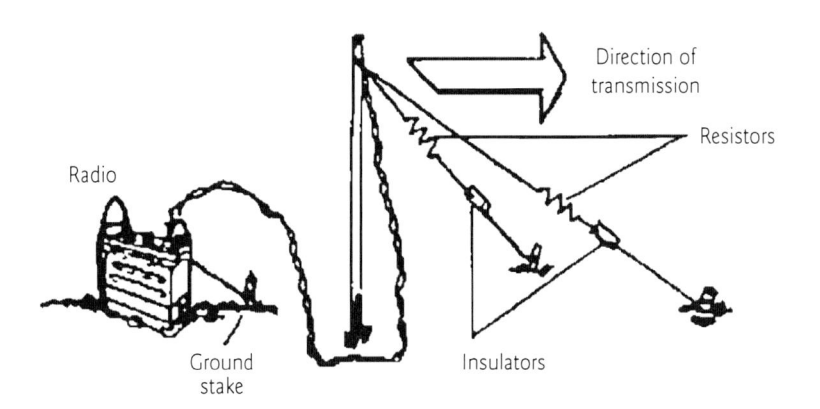

The sloping V antenna consists of two wires forming a V. The open end of the V is pointed toward the desired direction of transmission or reception. The apex of the V should be mounted 15 to 20 feet above the ground (although the antenna will work satisfactorily when as little as 3 or 4 feet off the ground). The antenna wires end with a noninductive terminating resistors at each end of the leg and a final insulator.

The angle between the two sloping wires that form the V depends on the length (in wavelengths) of the antenna. At 1 wavelength the wires have an optimal apex angle of 90 degrees, at 2 wavelengths 70 degrees, at 4 wavelengths 50 degrees, and at 10 wavelengths 33 degrees.

If you do the math for the 10-wavelength antenna, you will see that it is starting to get fairly large. You probably won't be setting up a 10-wavelength antenna, although this is not entirely outside the realm of possibility.

A general rule for antennas is that bigger is better than smaller, higher is better than lower, outside is better than inside, and cut to frequency is better than not.

CHAPTER 9

Covert Signals

DEAD DROP

A dead drop is a place where a message or a small package can be concealed until it can be recovered by another person. The dead drop differs from the cache in that the former is intended for short-term use, while the cache may hold items for years. Dead drops are used to pass material from one individual (or group) to another, while a cache is often used to support the same individual or group that established it. Finally, dead drops are usually much smaller than caches. Think of a dead drop as a covert mailbox.

A dead drop is used when you have people who are willing to support your evasion efforts, but with whom you may not wish to risk direct contact. The dead drop can be used to pass information and materials, as well as to receive information and materials. Dead drops have been used by intelligence services and special forces as a means of covert communication for decades. Let's take a look at how they work.

A dead drop consists of three parts: the concealment area, the "loaded signal," and the "recovered" signal.

The concealment area is where you hide the item(s) to be passed through the dead drop. The concealment area should be screened from direct observation, yet still be easily accessed. The dead drop must be able to be loaded and recovered rapidly. For the wilderness evader, dead drops will likely be on the edge of rural towns or perhaps in state or national park areas. The idea here is to have an area where someone supporting you can have easy access, yet where you also can gain access without exposing yourself in a town itself.

The loaded signal allows you to signal that something has been placed in the dead drop. You don't want to check the concealment area over and over again. In fact, you should only go near the concealment area when it is necessary to load something into or recover something from the dead drop. The loaded signal should be observable from a distance. As an example, the loaded signal might be a piece of colored cloth tied around the sign post at the intersection of Remote Highway and Rural Road. Someone supporting you from a town may spot this signal simply by driving through this intersection, and because this intersection is out of the way it can be seen from a distance (perhaps using binoculars).

The recovered signal allows the person who loaded the dead drop to know that whatever was loaded has been recovered, and by the proper person. There is always the possibility that the concealment area may be discovered by someone other than the intended recipient, and who will remove its contents. However, the only persons who know about the signals associated with the dead drop are those who are supposed to be using it. Thus a recovered signal confirms proper receipt of the contents of the dead drop.

It is important to be sure that the loaded and recovered signals are not located in the vicinity of the concealment area, and of course the signal itself should give no clue about the location of the concealment area. Additionally, as much as possible, the loaded and recovered signals should be in areas that can be reached in the normal course of your regular activities.

MAIL

As a general rule a wilderness evader will not have access to the postal service to send and receive mail. However, there may be times when you are able to briefly enter a small town or gain access to a mailbox located at some fairly remote location. You may want to send a letter to someone to assure him of your well-being, request some type of support, or accomplish some other purpose important enough for you to send the letter.

If you simply place your letter in an envelope, affix a stamp, and drop it in the mail, it will be delivered to the addressee. But the postmark will show the location from where the letter was mailed— and thus your location when you mailed it.

Some writers have suggested giving such a letter to a trucker traveling cross-country (or other long-distance traveler) and asking him to mail it from some distant location. However, as a wilderness evader you will not be in a position to meet many travelers or build enough of a friendship for them to help you out and mail the letter from the far side of the country.

You can however let the U.S. Postal Service do this for you. To get your mail postmarked from a distant city, first write your letter, place it in an envelope, and stick on a stamp as usual. Now, place this envelope into a second envelope addressed to the postmaster at some distant location, affix proper postage, and drop it in the mail. When the postmaster at the distant location receives the envelope containing your letter, he opens the outer envelope and now has a properly address letter with first-class postage on it. By law he can't open the inner envelope and must simply process the letter the same way as if you had handed it to him across the counter at the post office or dropped it into the mailbox on the corner. Your letter in the inner envelope is mailed to the addressee from whatever distant city you chose and has on it the postmark from that location.

I've tried this several times and have always received the inner envelope as if it had been mailed from a distant city. I have also spoken to various postmasters about this and asked whether this would raise any particular suspicion. It seems that this is actually a fairly common practice. Stamp collectors wanting a postmark on a particular stamp from a particular city (e.g., a Liberty Bell stamp and a Philadelphia postmark) will often use this same routine to obtain the postmark they seek. You may even want to include a brief note to the postmaster explaining that you want a postmark from his city. Generally, however, the note isn't necessary, and as long as the inner envelope contains no more than a letter you give the appearance of being in a location that you are not.

TRAIL MARKINGS

On occasion, it may be useful to mark a trail in a wilderness area. You may want to be sure of finding a specific place again, or more likely you want to leave a trail for someone else (but not your pursuers) to follow. The problem is to find a way of marking a trail that's apparent only to you or those you want to be able to find you and that is also not permanent.

The old method of blazing a trail by cutting marks in trees is a poor idea. Some have suggested marking trails with strips of survey tape (brightly colored plastic tape), and I have even heard one person suggest using business cards! These methods just litter the wilderness, and there is absolutely no excuse for such things.

When marking a trail, you should only use natural items (e.g., sticks, rocks). Your trail marking is not intended to be permanent. The old Boy Scout field books showed how to mark trails by stacking stones or tying bundles of grass together. These methods work well and do not damage the wilderness. You may want to adopt the methods from the Boy Scouts, though it is perhaps better to develop your own set of trail marking to use with friends.

Of course, it is just as easy to provide a grid coordinate or an azimuth route to anyone with basic navigation skills. Therefore, if you are planning to work with others in a remote area, make sure that everyone has some skill with map and compass.

CHAPTER 10

Navigation

Navigation is an essential skill for the wilderness evader. The ability to move along a given azimuth, to ascertain one's exact location on the ground, and to determine direction by expedient means greatly increase the chances of evading pursuit. This chapter is not an instruction manual for learning to use a map and compass. There are many such books currently available, and I make the assumption that you have some basic skill in this area already. You should have a top-quality compass in your kit and back it up with a second compass of at least very good quality (if not a copy of your primary compass).

If you should lose your primary compass and find that the needle has fallen off your backup compass, you must resort to expedient methods of determining direction. By "expedient methods," I mean some type of celestial navigation.

Celestial navigation gives you a different bearing than you get from magnetic navigation. This difference between "true" and "magnetic" is called *declination*. It is important to understand that declination varies depending on where you are. Because of this, almost all maps are oriented to true north, with the geographic North Pole at the top of the map. In the United States, declination varies from 25 degrees east declination in some parts of Alaska to 0 degrees declination in Wisconsin to 20 degrees west declination in Maine. It is important to know the declination in your planned evasion area.

SHADOW-TIP METHOD

To determine direction using the shadow-tip method, place a stick about 1 yard long into the ground so that it stands straight up. Take a second small stick or a stone and mark the location of the tip of the shadow cast by the stick. Wait 20 or 30 minutes and you will see that the shadow has moved because of the rotation of the earth (the sun's movement from east to west). Mark the new location of the tip of the shadow. Draw a line between the two marks—this is an east-west line. The first mark is always westerly and the second easterly. Stand with your left foot on the first mark and your right foot on the second mark and you are facing north.

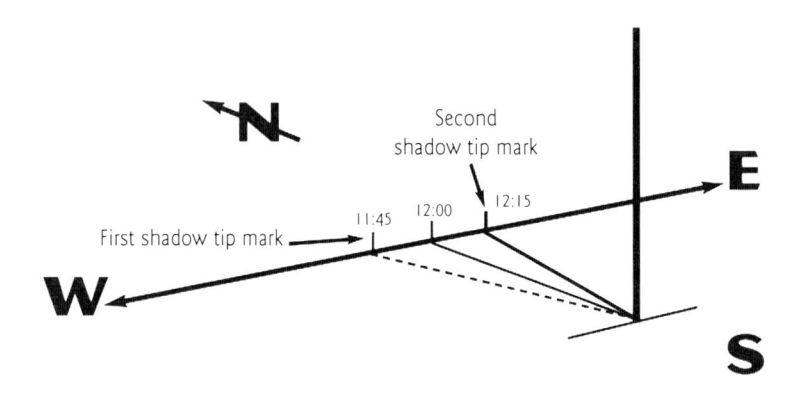

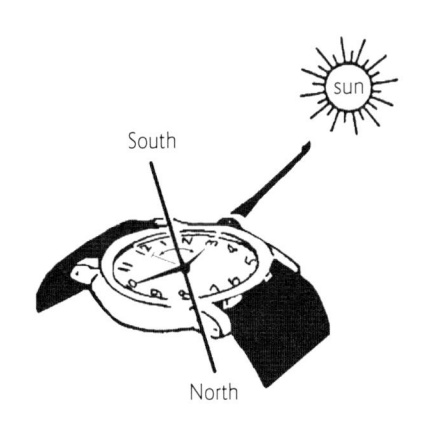

WATCH METHOD

You can also determine direction by using your watch. Hold your watch horizontally and point the hour hand toward the sun. A line bisecting the angle between the hour hand and the 12 o'clock position on your watch is a north-south line, with south being closest to the 12 o'clock position. To be accurate your watch must be set to local standard time, not daylight savings time. If your watch is set to daylight savings time, use the point midway between the hour hand and the 1 o'clock position to determine the north-south line. The farther you are away from the equator, the greater the accuracy of this technique.

Another interesting use for this method is that it can be used with a compass to set your watch if it has stopped. Simply reverse the watch method for finding direction. First, find true south (magnetic south and adjust for declination). Now adjust your watch so that the halfway point between 12 o'clock and the hour hand of your watch pointing at the sun lies directly on this line. Your watch is now set to within a few minutes of the correct local standard time.

POLAR STAR

Polaris, the Polar Star, or the North Star as the name implies, is directly over the North Pole. This star is constant and does not vary its position in the sky, thus allowing anyone who can locate the North Star to determine direction. Anyone who spends time outdoors at night quickly learns to locate the North Star. Someone unfamiliar with the night sky may however have difficulty locating the North Star or may confuse it with other brighter objects in the sky.

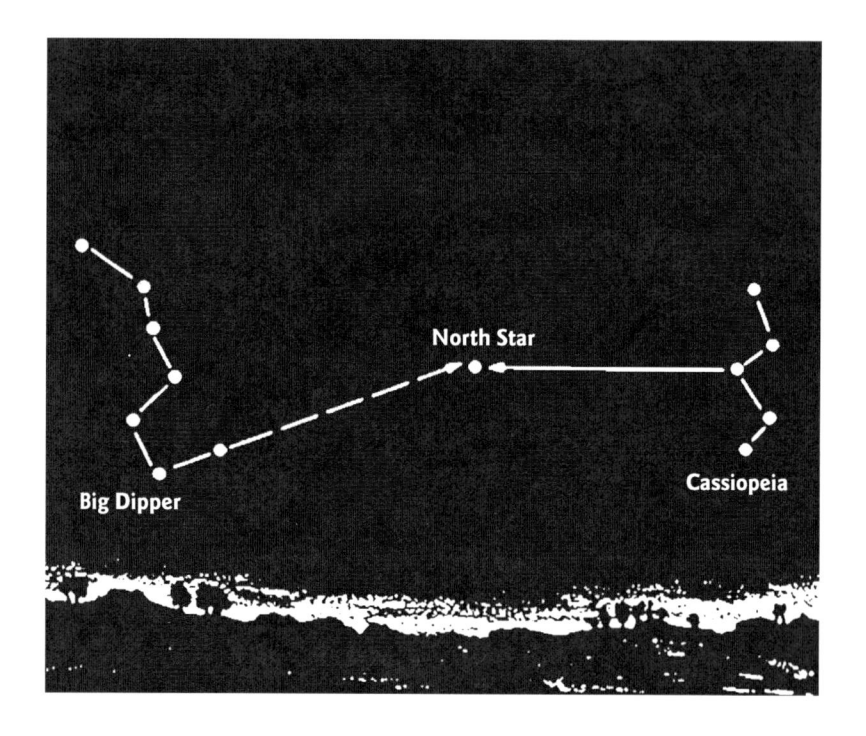

[Figure: Big Dipper, North Star, and Cassiopeia]

In the northern sky the two most easily recognized constellations are the Big Dipper and Cassiopeia. Neither of these constellations ever sets, so they are always visible in a clear night sky. Although the North Star is not part of either of these constellations (it is part of the Little Dipper) you can use the Big Dipper and Cassiopeia to easily locate the North Star. The Big Dipper is directly opposite Cassiopeia in the sky, and both of these constellations rotate around the North Star in a counterclockwise direction. To locate the North Star using the Big Dipper, locate the two stars on the outer lip of the dipper. Draw a line through these two stars and extend it five times the distance between the stars themselves and you will find the North Star on the line. Now locate Cassiopeia, which consists of five stars that look like a "W" in the sky, which is opposite the Big Dipper. Draw a line straight out from the center star of Cassiopeia and you will locate the North Star.

MAKING A COMPASS

It is possible to make a compass by magnetizing a piece of ferrous metal. For example, a needle can be magnetized by stroking it in one direction with a piece of silk or a magnet if you have one. It is also possible to magnetize a piece of metal by rubbing it repeatedly through your hair in one direction. Be sure that you stroke the needle in one direction only.

A battery of at least 2 volts and a coil of wire can be used to magnetize a needle also. Attach the ends of the coil of wire to the battery terminals and then insert one end of the needle into the center of the coil. Be careful not to let the needle actually touch the coil of wire or it will mess up your magnetization.

Once you have a magnetized needle, float it in still water on a leaf or thin piece of wood. The magnetized end will point to magnetic north. If you don't have a needle, but have some other piece of ferrous metal, you can magnetize one end and hang it from its center point by a thin thread or long hair so that it swings freely. The magnetized end will swing to point north.

CHAPTER 11

Firearms for Survival

This chapter is not intended as a definitive assessment of firearms. That is beyond the scope of this book, and there are many fine books already out that do just that. After reading this chapter, if you desire more information about firearms in general or any specific models, check Paladin's selection in the firearms and combat shooting categories of its catalog.

THE UBIQUITOUS .22

Perhaps the greatest advantage of the .22 is its universality. Every store selling firearms seems to have some sort of .22 rifle or pistol, and anywhere you can purchase ammunition you almost certainly can find some type of .22 ammunition.

A small .22 rifle and a couple hundred rounds of ammunition take up little space in your pack and can more than make up for the little weight it adds by keeping fresh meat in the pot.

I strongly recommend the inclusion of a compact .22 rifle in your survival or evasion kit. A number of quality .22-caliber rifles are available today, but for our purposes we will consider only those compact enough to be carried disassembled inside a rucksack. Although it is true that any rifle can be disassembled given the right tools, only those rifles specifically designed to be dissembled, or that can be disassembled without tools, will be discussed here.

When discussing survival rifles, there are at least as many opinions regarding what makes the ideal survival rifle as there are people willing to discuss the topic. One of the main differences of opinion is between those who recommend a .22-caliber rifle and those who favor a major-caliber centerfire rifle.

The main argument in favor of a large-caliber rifle is that it can be used to take large game, which yields much more meat per shot. Furthermore, a large-caliber rifle allows you to use the rifle in a combat or self-defense role. The argument in favor of the .22-caliber rifle is weight: a small .22 and 500 rounds of ammunition probably weigh less than the major-caliber rifle itself. Plus, you are much more likely to have the opportunity to shoot small game (e.g., squirrels, rabbits) than larger game (e.g., deer or elk). With careful shooting a .22-caliber rifle can take deer and large game, and in a self-defense situation the same careful shooting can cause a pursuer to give up the chase.

There is merit to both sides of this argument. I believe the advantage of light weight and almost universal availability is a very persuasive argument for choosing a .22-caliber rifle. However, a full-size rifle is perhaps more than we need in a .22. A handgun with an 8- or 10-inch barrel and fitted with a detachable shoulder stock would be ideal in a survival situation. Unfortunately, abusive government regulations make such a setup illegal. The next best option is a .22-caliber rifle specifically designed as a "survival rifle."

There is a handful of rifles designed to be broken down and carried in a rucksack or survival kit that I recommend. These rifles are as follows:

FIREARMS FOR SURVIVAL

- Springfield M6 Scout
- Charter Arms/U.S. Henry AR7
- Marlin 70P Papoose
- New England Firearms SS Youth Model
- Ruger 10/22 Takedown

You can find out more about these rifles in the catalogs and on the Web pages of the companies that manufacture them. Major gun stores probably carry most of these survival rifles, allowing you the opportunity to compare them in person and decide which is best for you.

My personal favorite is the Springfield M6 Scout. It has the advantage of a .410 shotgun combined with the versatility of a .22-caliber. Others may prefer the advantage of rapid follow-up shots offered by rifles such as the Marlin 70P. I strongly believe that the inclusion of a survival rifle is important, but the specific rifle to include in your kit comes down to personal preference.

CB CAPS AND BB CAPS

Since you are carrying a .22 rifle, you need some ammunition to go with it. In addition to standard .22 Long Rifle ammunition, I also recommend that you include some CB or BB caps in your kit.

Although .22 CB ammunition (CB caps) should be in everyone's field gear collection, for some reason many people don't even know they exist. The CB cap is a short, low-power .22-caliber round. It is a 29-grain bullet, fired at around 700 to 800 feet per second. It doesn't have a lot of power or range, but it has the advantage of being very quiet. The report of a CB cap is no louder than that of a pellet gun, maybe even less so. Fired outside a building, the CB cap is completely inaudible to anyone inside and is unlikely to be detected outside by anyone several yards away.

CB caps won't cycle a semiautomatic firearm, so they must be loaded one at a time. I have had no problem feeding them in my Marlin Model 81TS, which is a tube-fed, bolt-action rifle. They work just fine in revolvers and single-shot rifles. As noted, the CB cap is of very low power, but it still has enough to kill such small game as rabbits and squirrels.

Because of its low noise the CB cap can be used to shoot more than one animal in a group. A standard .22 when fired will frighten other animals into running for cover—not so, however, with the CB cap. Using a single-shot rifle and CB caps I have been able to take five rabbits in an open field before they realized they were being hunted.

Even smaller than the CB cap is the BB cap. This is a 17-grain lead BB fired from a short .22 cartridge. They have even less power than the CB cap and for all practical purposes make no noise. I don't like BB caps because the power of these rounds is less than that of a good-quality pellet rifle. I have also found that the accuracy of the BB cap is not enough to ensure head shots on such game as rabbits and body shots may be not be enough to stop or kill game. However, you may find that they fill your particular needs better than the CB caps.

CB caps cost about $4.00 per box of 100. BB caps cost about $13.00 per box of 100. It is definitely worth having a box of CB caps available for those times when a quiet shot or two is needed. I consider BB caps very specialized ammunition, to be used only when noise is the primary consideration.

GENERAL-PURPOSE RIFLE

A general-purpose rifle is one that can do at least reasonably well all things expected of a rifle. Of course, no rifle is the perfect choice for every situation, so you need a rifle that gives you the widest possible number of options. A rifle makes a man master of his surroundings. It must be capable of striking a decisive blow on man, beast, or machine at any distance from which the shooter can clearly define his target.

In addition to being powerful enough, the caliber of your general-purpose rifle must be generally available. The ".750 Belch-Fire Back Blast Ultra Magnum" may be your idea of the ultimate rifle, but if you can't get ammunition for it, it's just a big unwieldy stick. Taking availability into consideration, I favor the .308 Winchester (7.62 NATO) because of the almost universal availability of ammunition from military surplus. Yes, other calibers may offer a slight ballistic advantage, but this advantage seems insignificant when weighed against other factors.

There is, however, a disadvantage to any rifle: it is difficult to conceal and when carried openly tends to attract attention. In remote areas this may not be a problem, but it must be considered in any area where there is the potential for encountering other people.

HANDGUNS

Is a handgun necessary? For a person alone in the wilderness I believe it is. You have only yourself to rely on for your own safety. Even if you have a way to call for help and there is someone ready to respond, the problem will likely have ended one way or another before help arrives. This same principle applies even in the largest cities. Calling 911 usually does nothing to prevent an attack; it just dispatches someone to fill out the reports, bandage wounds, or zip up the body bag. Of course, in the wilderness calling 911 is a moot point because it simply isn't available.

Compared with a rifle, any handgun is woefully underpowered and inaccurate, but it has the advantage of being readily available at all times. Whether you are cooking a meal, chopping wood, gathering plants, or doing pretty much anything else, your handgun can be securely holstered on your hip. If you travel into a town, a handgun can rest concealed beneath your coat.

The debate over what type of handgun to carry for personal protection is not something that can be resolved in the pages of this book. It all comes down to making an informed choice and selecting something that{s right for you.

For use in the wilderness, I recommend that you carry a large-caliber handgun. This means .45 ACP, .45 Colt, .44 Special or Magnum, and maybe .357 Magnum. You want a handgun capable of halting the attack of an aggressive animal at close range. Whether this animal is on two legs or four, you want all the edge that you can get to stop the attack, or at least to fight your way to your rifle (which should be close by).

SHOTGUNS

I am not a big fan of shotguns for survival or evasion purposes. They do offer a degree of versatility when combined with a rifle (such as the Springfield M6 Scout or the Savage Model 24) but generally are not worth the size and weight. Shotgun shells tend to be bulky and offer limited range when compared with rifle, or even pistol, rounds used by a skilled marksman.

CHAPTER 12

Primitive Weapons

Few people think of primitive weapons as being of much value any more. After all, we have modern firearms, they say. Didn't we just finish discussing the importance of at least having a .22-caliber survival rifle in our kit? Yes, firearms are important, but they may break, ammunition may run out, or the noise of a gunshot can't be risked.

THROWING STICK

The throwing stick (also called a rabbit stick) is one of the first primitive weapons you'll want to make. Think of a throwing stick as a boomerang that doesn't return.

Of course, any stick can be thrown, but by shaping the stick properly you have a much more effective weapon. By flattening and beveling a curved stick you get greater gyroscopic stability from the spin during the throw, as well as more lift based on the Bernoulli principle.

The throwing stick is thrown with a side-arm motion, imparting spin to the stick as it is thrown. A properly made throwing stick is very effective in killing small game, such as rabbits or birds on the ground. The throwing stick can also be thrown into a flock of birds in flight with a fair degree of success. Larger animals may be stunned with a throwing stick, but generally it will not be successful against them. However, aborigines in Australia are known to have killed animals as large as kangaroos with the throwing stick (boomerang). Some reports state that the throwing stick is effective at ranges up to 200 yards. I suppose that this is possible, but I have never had much success with a throwing stick beyond 40 or 50 yards. With practice, however, you may be able to achieve better results.

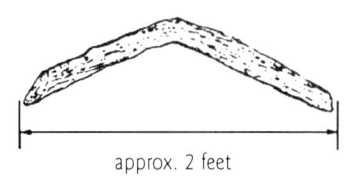

SLING

Anyone who attended Sunday school as a child is familiar with the sling, the weapon with which David killed Goliath. It was also a weapon used with great effect by ancient armies. The sling is nothing more than two cords with a pouch at the center to hold a stone to be thrown. The sling is easy to make, lightweight and easy to carry, and extremely effective in practiced hands. A sling can throw a half-pound rock over 100 yards with relative ease, and with practice you can consistently hit a target the size of a #10 coffee can at 20 or 25 yards. This is better than some people can do with a pistol.

Centrifugal force holds the stone in the pouch of the sling as it is swung and adds power to the throw when one of the cords is released.

Mastering the use of the sling takes a bit of practice, and this is its primary disadvantage. You cannot put a sling together today and expect to use it for hunting tomorrow. If you plan on using a sling as a survival weapon, I suggest you make one now and learn how to use it. Then you can either carry it with you or make one when needed, but either way you have the skill to use it.

PRIMITIVE WEAPONS

To make a sling you'll need two cords about 2 1/2 feet each in length and a piece of leather or other strong material about 4 inches by 7 inches to make the sling pouch. Attach the cords to each end of the pouch. In the end of one of the cords tie a small loop that will fit over two fingers. If using leather for a sling pouch, you can soak it in water and then tie it tightly around a rock of the basic size and shape you plan to throw. This forms the pouch so that it holds the stone a little better, but it is not absolutely necessary to make a good sling.

The best stones to throw with a sling are about the size of a small chicken egg and should be fairly smooth and round (or egg shaped). To throw the stone, place it in the sling pouch and slip the loop in the cord over one or two fingers. Adjust the second cord so that the pouch hangs evenly. The stone is thrown by either using an overhand whiplike motion or by whirling the sling above your head and releasing the free cord (the cord without the loop around your fingers) toward the target.

BOLA

Another weapon useful for hunting small game and birds is the bola. The bola is made by attaching weights (such as rocks in cloth pouches) to the end of cords. The weights are spun about at the end of the cords, and the whole device is thrown at the target. Centrifugal force causes the weights to spin at the end of the cords, which entangle the target that is then struck by the spinning weights.

To make a bola you need three weights and two strong cords. The first cord should be between 5 and 6 feet long. The second cord is half the length of the first cord. Attach a weight to each end of the longest cord. After the weights are attached, tie the short cord to the exact center of the long cord with a knot that won't slip. I find it best to tie an overhand loop in the center of the long cord and tie the short cord to the loop. Now at the free end of the short cord attach your third weight.

To use the bola, grasp the weight on the short cord and spin the bola in a circular motion above your head. Throw the bola directly at your target. The spinning motion of the bola causes the weights to spread out to the length of the cord holding them together.

Some advocate holding the bola by the center knot when spinning it prior to the throw, but I find this causes the weights to bunch up rather than spreading out during flight.

The bola is simple to build and seems to work fairly well when thrown into flocks of flying birds. I have had no success using the bola on such small game as rabbits and squirrels, but you may have better luck if you practice enough.

THROWING KNIFE

A knife can be thrown and used as an effective hunting weapon. Such notable knife experts as Harry K. McEvoy and Blackie Collins have reported killing game as large as wild pigs with throwing knives. It is important to note that any knife can be thrown, but the most effective throwing knives are those specifically designed for that purpose.

You should not use your primary knife for throwing. The risks of losing your knife generally outweigh any advantage you may gain by throwing it. On the other hand, having a throwing knife (which is also usable for other purposes) provides another means of taking game.

The throwing knife you choose should have some weight to it. I recommend a minimum of 1/2 pound. Avoid the lightweight sets of throwing knives. Even if you get a good hit on your target, you still need some weight behind the knife to get sufficient penetration to kill your target. I prefer the Cold Steel True Flight Thrower, 10 3/4 inches overall and weighing in at 8 1/2 ounces. The True Flight Thrower also has an edge that can be sharpened (allowing it to be used as a utility knife) and a cord-wrapped handle to keep it from slipping in your hand. I have also had good success with Gil Hibben's throwing knives.

To be able to use a throwing knife for killing game requires practice, lots of practice. I recommend that you practice throwing your knife 100 times per day, every day for a month before even considering using it for hunting. When throwing your knife, you must be able to judge distance accurately and know that when you throw it it will stick point first into the target. We all miss from time to time, but with practice you can be sure of sticking your knife far more often than you miss.

ATLATL

The atlatl is a spear thrower or, more appropriately, a dart thrower. An atlatl dart looks like a large arrow or perhaps a spear with fletching. An atlatl dart varies in length from 5 to 8 feet, and is somewhere around 1/2 inch in diameter. A point or blade is added to the front end of the dart, and fletching (feathers, vanes) are added to the rear of the dart to help stabilize it in flight. The atlatl itself is a narrow board, around 2 or 3 feet in length, with a small projection or nub on one end to connect with the butt end of the dart. The dart is accelerated from that end (just like a bow and arrow). When accelerated from the rear, the dart flexes and moves rapidly away from the atlatl. The mass of the dart and the atlatl accelerating that dart determine the rate at which this energy is stored and released.

To use, place the dart on the atlatl with the rear of the dart connecting with the projection on the end of the atlatl. Using an overhand-pitching type of motion, throw the dart forward, following through so that the atlatl continues to accelerate the dart from the end throughout the throw. It doesn't take much effort to become proficient with the atlatl and dart. The atlatl can be used for anything that can be hunted with a bow and arrow. Its effective range is similar to that of a bow and arrow. The record distance for throwing an atlatl dart is 848.5 feet, set in Aurora, Colorado, in 1995.

There is even an association of atlatl users. If you are interested in more information about the atlatl, write to the World Atlatl Association, Inc., P.O. Box 56, Ocotillo, California 92259.

BOW AND ARROW

The bow and arrow is perhaps the first primitive weapon to come to mind, and it is certainly the one that has carried over to the greatest extent today. Bows of the finest quality can be made by hand, using just the simplest of tools, but this is the art of the master bowyer. For our purposes here, we'll concentrate on simpler bows that are suitable for survival purposes.

The most basic bow and arrow you can make is simply a stick flexed to keep tension on a string and a fairly straight stick. This enables you to launch a stick (arrow) along a fairly straight line over a distance of several feet. If you cut a straight sapling or reed (such as cattail) for an arrow, the thickest (heaviest) end should be used as the tip of the arrow. Although this will work, and may be suitable for taking a rabbit or similar game, you can make a much better bow.

To make a bow of good quality, first begin by finding a straight sapling, about 2 inches in diameter and as free as possible of knots and branches. Some of the best woods for making bows are yew, ash, and mountain mahogany, but any type of wood can be used. You obviously can only use the wood available in your area.

Cut the sapling to be used for the bow stave and remove the bark (prepare a couple of acceptable saplings so you have a spare). Once you have removed the bark, let the stave dry for a day or two.

Next you must determine the natural bend of the stave. This is done by placing one end of the stave on the ground, supporting the top end of the stave, and applying pressure to the center. This will cause the stave to turn and flex along its natural bend. The curve of the stave facing away from you will become the back (outside curve) of the completed bow.

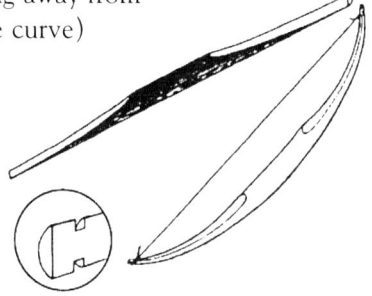

Now begin to shape the bow by gently tapering the stave from the center to the ends. Work on one limb of the bow at a time. Complete the top limb and then begin work on the lower limb of the bow. The bow should remain round as you shape it so that it makes a smooth taper to the end of each limb.

Once you have tapered both limbs of the bow, you flatten the belly of the bow (the inside of the curve of the bow) to increase its flexibility along its entire length. Don't get carried away here; you want to increase the flexibility of the bow, but don't thin it so much that it becomes weak.

Now that you have the stave shaped, notch each end of the bow to receive the bowstring. The string can be permanently tied to one end of the bow, and a loop placed in the other end of the string so that it slips securely into the notches when the bow is flexed.

To preserve the wood of your new bow, rub it thoroughly with animal fat or grease. You can save the fat from meats that you cook. Repeat this process from time to time to keep the wood supple. When the bow is not in use, it should be stored unstrung.

Arrows

Now that you have a bow, you need some arrows to shoot from it. Making arrows is not particularly complicated, but you must begin with shafts that are reasonably straight. Find several new saplings that are straight and without many branches or knots, or you can also use reeds, such as cattails, as the basis for your arrow shafts. Collect several shafts for your arrows and tie them together in bundles and let them dry for a couple days. This helps to straighten the shafts. Shafts can also be straightened by rubbing their bent areas with grease and straightening them over a fire.

If the shafts taper at all, the larger end of the shaft becomes the tip of the arrow, and the thinner end becomes the tail. It is best to make arrows of a uniform diameter, but there is often a slight taper to arrows made in a survival situation. It is possible to make arrows by simply sharpening the larger end of the shaft and carving a notch into the thinner end. Without fletching, these arrows are effective out to several yards. Fletching increases range and stability and is made by splitting large feathers and binding them to the arrow shaft and then trimming them to shape. Pine pitch or glue made from animal bones can be used to secure the fletching to the shaft.

You probably also want to add a better point for hunting larger game. To do this (especially when using reeds for shafts), make a fore-shaft out of wood and harden it by fire. You may also chip stone arrowheads and bind them to the fore-shafts of your arrows. A very effective arrowhead can be cut from the lid of a tin can. These are thin and lightweight and can be sharpened to a razor's edge. When bound to your arrow shaft the tin arrowhead works much like a commercial broad-head arrow.

CHAPTER 13

Shelters

For the wilderness evader, shelters may be categorized into temporary shelters used en route to your base camp (and during other travel) and the semipermanent shelter you establish as your base camp.

BASE CAMP

Your base camp is the area where you'll stay once you have evaded pursuers and disappeared into a remote wilderness area. Your base camp becomes your home, so it should be more than a simple lean-to or tarp. It should be a semipermanent structure. Assuming that you have the material, a hard-sided tent, or a tepee may be sufficient. U.S. soldiers have been deployed to such places as Bosnia and lived in tents for 6 months to a year. However, these military tents are not something that can be carried into an area in your backpack.

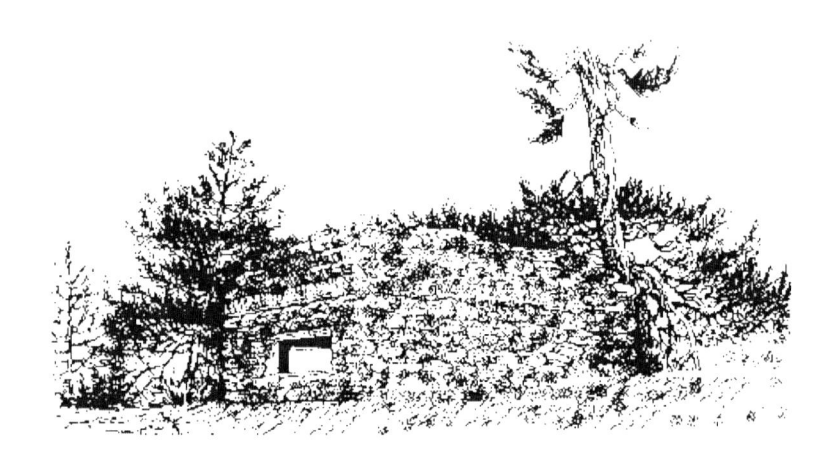

Ideally, your base camp is constructed of natural material and built so that it blends in with the natural surroundings.

In a remote area you may be able to build a log cabin into the side of a hill. However, even if the finished product blends into the area fairly well, the felling of trees to build the cabin will make the area clearly visible, especially from the air.

If there are numerous saplings growing in the area, you can build woven brush walls (waffle). When these walls are completed and packed with mud (daub) they become very sturdy, forming a waffle-and-daub structure.

To build a woven brush wall you begin by burying several poles in the ground so that they stand vertically, approximately 20 inches apart. The base of each pole should be put about 1 foot into the ground to provide stability. After the poles are all in place to establish the framework of your shelter, weave additional saplings and brush horizontally between the poles to form the walls. The tops of the vertical poles may

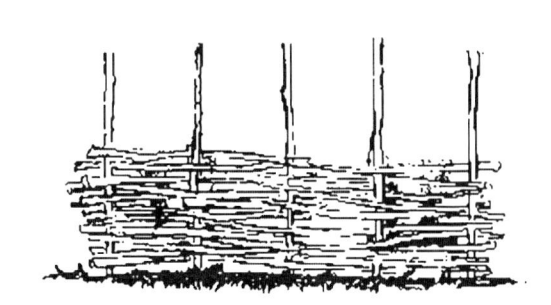

SHELTERS

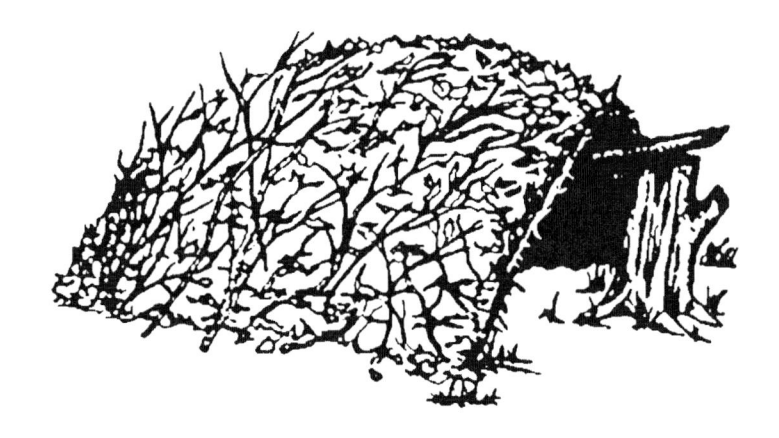

be curved inward to meet and form the roof of the shelter, or a heavier ridgepole and frame may be used to support a separate roof. Once complete, the walls should be packed with mud to close gaps in the brush and make the walls more solid.

A similar shelter is the debris shelter. This shelter is made by angling a long ridgepole from a vertical support. The vertical support can be a tree, tall stump, or the wall of a cliff. Once the ridgepole is in place, angle additional poles off the ridgepole and cover the entire framework with debris. The ridgepole needs to be strong and well secured in place. I like to bury one end of the pole and nail the other end firmly into the vertical support. The supporting framework should be nailed or lashed to the ridgepole. Then the entire framework is covered with debris, such as brush, bark, and dirt.

When constructing a base camp shelter, there are some general considerations to keep in mind.

- Perhaps most important for the wilderness evader, the shelter must blend in with the natural surroundings. A shelter that stands out will certainly attract attention and be discovered by any search. On the other hand, a shelter that blends in with the surrounding may not be seen even when someone passes very near it.

- The shelter should have a low silhouette. This goes along with blending in with the surroundings. Your shelter should not be built on a hilltop or on the crest of a ridge where it is silhouetted against the sky. Where possible, build your shelter about 75 to 100 feet up the hill from a valley floor, but below the crest of the ridge.
- The shelter should be of irregular shape. Avoid sharp angles and lines on the outside of the completed shelter. A shelter constructed from natural materials and built into a hillside or natural deadfall usually accomplishes this.
- The shelter should be small. You are building a shelter that is basically one room. It should have room enough for a bed, an area to sit, a place to store some gear and enough room to stand up, but you are not building an eight-room house. Think of the camper mounted on the back of a pick-up truck as the basic size for your base camp shelter. The smaller shelter is easier to heat and maintain, and meets the first requirement of blending in with the surroundings much more easily than a larger shelter.

An excellent guide to building wilderness shelters is D.C. Beard's book, *Shelters, Shacks, and Shanties*. Originally published in 1914, this book is again available from Loompanics Unlimited in Port Townsend, Washington.

TEMPORARY CAMPSITES

When on the way to your base camp or traveling in the backwoods for other purposes, you'll have to stop from time to time and make camp. Temporary campsites should be kept as simple as possible. This may mean nothing more than spreading your bedroll out on the ground and going to sleep, but usually you'll want a little bit more.

I recommend carrying a small "backpacker type" of tent or a tarp to erect a shelter. Along with a sleeping bag or warm blankets, this can keep you warm and dry overnight. The advantage of a tent or tarp is that it allows you to quickly set up a shelter without disturbing the natural surroundings. Your tent or tarp should be a color that blends in with the environment, such as green, brown, and gray. A couple of military shelter halves work well, but since they are made of canvas they are a little heavier than nylon and other lightweight fabrics. A tent can be easily made from military ponchos, which are the same general size as the shelter halves but significantly lighter. The Austrian army employs a basic arrangement whereby four men use their ponchos to make a tepee-like shelter for overnight bivouac.

A small multifuel camp stove (see Chapter 14) can preclude the need to light a campfire at a temporary site, although a small fire with a hobo stove leaves little trace.

The basic idea with your temporary camp is to keep it small and disturb the area as little as possible. Your temporary camp allows you to get out of the elements, get some rest and a warm meal, and then move on.

SECURITY OF YOUR CAMP

Once you have your base camp established, you have to consider security. In the backwoods you are completely responsible for your own security. As noted earlier, dialing 911 is absolutely useless, even assuming that you had something to dial it from in the first place. Never think that you are in an area so remote that you'll never be found. If you made it to your base camp, others can too.

The best way of protecting yourself is to be armed and aware. This applies not only in the wilderness, but anywhere and at any time. A man who is armed and aware of what is going on around him is very difficult to harm. Yes, it is possible to overcome him through superior numbers or firepower, and a sniper may kill him from a distance, but generally he is master of his own destiny.

One of the best aids for awareness is an early warning device or alarm. An interesting alarm, the Hunter and Camper Alert is made by the Driveway Alarm Company <http://www.drivewayalarm.com>. This unit has a remote sensor and a pager-like receiver. Simply set the receiver to sound a tone or vibrate whenever something passes in front of the sensor and place the detector on the approach to your camp.

Along this same line, tripwires connected to flares or other alerting devices can be used to warn that someone's approaching the camp. These alerting devices can be easily manufactured at home or purchased at military surplus stores. Devices designed to fire a 12-gauge blank shell are readily available. The devices can also be loaded with a tear gas shell to repel anyone approaching your camp. Another advantage of the 12-gauge alerting devices is that they work well to scare bears and other wild animals away from your camp and food supplies. It's important to be sure that these kind of devices contain only a blank shell or tear gas. The last thing you want to do is load the device with a shot shell and then have a wounded bear in the area of your camp.

There may be times when you wish to determine whether someone has been into your stuff. An example might be tying shut the door to a shelter when you leave and being able to tell whether someone has been inside while you were gone. Of course, someone could simply retie the cord, and assuming other things are not disturbed, you might never know that anyone had been in you place. The next time you use cord to secure something, use a "thief's knot." The thief's knot looks just like a square knot when the ends of the cord are covered. Almost everyone will mistake the thief's knot for a square knot and will tie a square knot when retying the cord. The difference between the thief's knot and the square knot is in the position of the ends of the cord. When you tie a square knot the ends of the cord are always on the same side of the knot. With the thief's knot, however, the ends of the cord are on opposite sides of the knot.

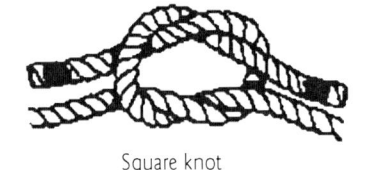

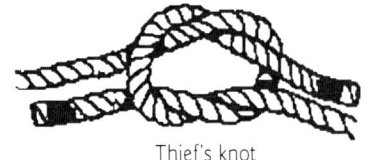

Square knot

Thief's knot

SHELTERS

To tie the thief's knot, form a loop with one of the cords. Thread the other end of the cord through the loop, around and under the loop, and back through the loop itself. This places the ends of the cord on opposite sides of the knot.

The thief's knot does nothing to keep someone from getting into your stuff, but it will almost always reveal if someone has entered your property surreptitiously.

Chapter 14

Fire

Fire is essential in any wilderness environment. It provides warmth and comfort, allows food to be cooked and water to be purified, and gives light at night. In many survival situations fire can be used to attract attention and signal for help. For the wilderness evader, however, attracting the attention of others is not what you want to do. Does this mean that you go without fire? It may be necessary to forgo a fire on some occasions, but there are clearly ways to have fire without attracting the attention of every person in the county.

The first consideration when building a fire that will not attract attention is to keep it small. You don't need a bonfire to cook your food and give you warmth. In fact a smaller fire lets you sit closer, taking greater advantage of its warmth. Small fires also use less fuel, meaning that you have to gather less wood.

Even a small fire can attract attention if built or located improperly. Your fires in an evasion scenario should be small, built with dry wood to limit smoke, and, where possible, built beneath overhanging tree branches to disperse any smoke that may rise. In remote areas smoky fires tend to get reported as possible forest fires, resulting in someone showing up to check things out.

HOBO STOVE

One method of maintaining a small fire is by using a "hobo stove." A hobo stove is simply a can with an opening cut in its side to feed fuel to the fire and holes punched around the top of the can to provide ventilation. The top of the can becomes a heating or cooking surface. Because the fire is under the can it is somewhat shielded from view.

DAKOTA HOLE

Another method of building a hidden fire is to build it below the surface of the ground. This type of fire is called a "Dakota hole.". To build a Dakota hole fire, first dig a hole in the ground about 1 foot deep and 1 foot in diameter. You build your fire in the

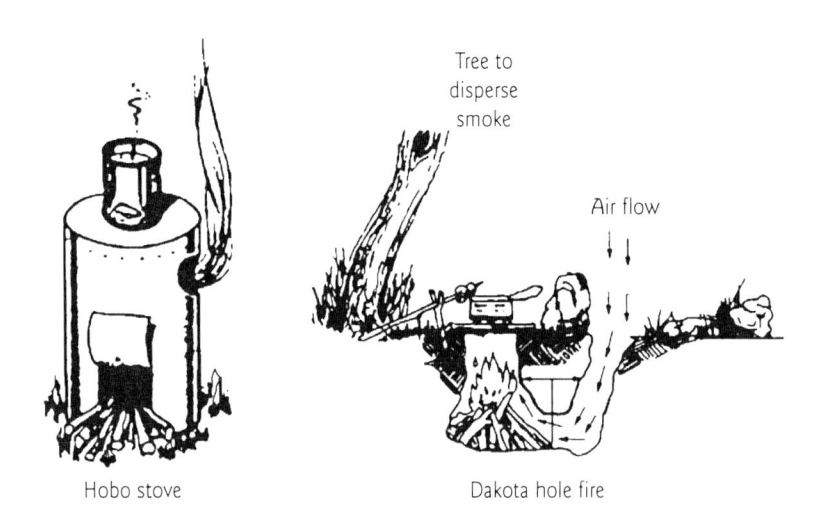

Hobo stove

Dakota hole fire

FIRE

bottom of this hole. However, a fire built in a hole doesn't burn very well because it lacks a good flow of oxygen. To provide oxygen for your fire, dig a second hole angling down to the bottom of the first. If the Dakota hole is situated so that any smoke is filtered through overhanging tree branches, the fire will be very difficult to detect from a distance. Another advantage of the this fire is that by filling in the holes before you leave the area you hide the fact there was any fire in the area at all.

Once a fire has been built, letting it die to a bed of hot coals is usually better for cooking. It provides a more even heat and has very little smoke. Adding a piece of dry hardwood from time to time keeps the fire small and continues to build on the bed of coals.

SOLAR OVEN

In addition to cooking over a fire or bed of coals you can construct a solar oven to cook your food. The solar oven is made from cardboard and aluminum foil. It reflects the heat of the sun to a center area, where you set a pan containing the food you want to cook.

To make a solar oven, begin with a cardboard box. Cut along the seams of the box so that it forms a "T" shape when laid flat. You may want to reinforce the seams and edges with a strong tape at this time, but it isn't necessary.

Next cut pieces of heavy-duty aluminum foil to completely line what will become the inside of the solar oven. Aluminum foil usually has a bright reflective side and a duller side. Be sure that the reflective side is out when placing the foil on the cardboard.

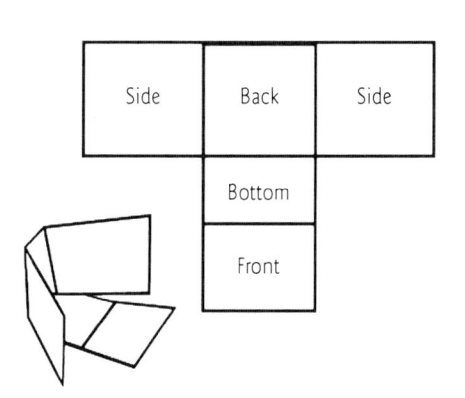

Now place a coat of glue on the cardboard and carefully put the aluminum foil in place. Make sure the reflective side is up and keep the foil as smooth as possible as you place it onto the cardboard. When gluing the foil to the cardboard, be sure that you flex the cardboard or split the aluminum foil at the seams. If you don't, the foil will be too tight when you try to fold the cardboard after the glue dries. I generally let the foil dry flat and then use a sharp knife to carefully split the foil along the seams.

This completes your solar oven. You'll need a pot in which to cook your food in the solar oven. The pot should be flat black to absorb the reflected heat of the sun. I use a coffee can that I spray-painted flat black, but any black pot should work.

I have seen solar ovens sold commercially for more than $100 that are little more than what you can make. The commercial versions don't seem to work any better than this version, which you can make for $5 or less. Now that you have your solar oven completed, it's time to cook some food.

Place your food in the black pot and set in on the bottom of your solar oven. Now angle the back, sides, and front of the oven so that the rays of the sun are reflected toward the center of the oven and onto the pot containing your food.

On a sunny day the temperature in the solar oven easily reaches 200 degrees Fahrenheit, and at times much hotter. The temperature in the solar oven depends on the intensity of the sun, the surrounding air temperature, and whether there is any wind to carry away the heat. You can limit the effects of the wind by including some oven bags with your solar oven. Although not absolutely necessary, oven bags are clear plastic bags designed to cook various types of meat (e.g., turkey, roast beef) in the oven. The bags hold in the natural juices of the meat and make cleanup easier. Don't use regular plastic bags; they will melt. By placing your black cooking pot in the bag you limit the effect of wind on your solar oven.

The solar oven slowly cooks your food and keeps it hot throughout the day. Just remember to rotate the oven to keep it facing the sun throughout the day.

CHAPTER 15

Camouflage

Simply defined, camouflage is the disguising or hiding of an object to make its detection more difficult. When we think of camouflage we make think of military uniforms or maybe hunters' attire. These are examples of camouflage, but it is important to understand just what camouflage is supposed to disguise.

To help remember all the aspects of camouflage, some people use the mnemonic S7M: shape, shadow, shine, silhouette, surface, sound, smell, and movement. Let's take a look at each to see how they apply to camouflage.

SHAPE

Shape is perhaps the basis for our identification of objects. When we see a person at a distance we may not be able to recognize him as a specific individual, but the basic shape easily signals a human.

SHADOW

Shadows may be broken into two categories: cast and deep. Cast shadows are most familiar. A person hiding behind a tree may be easily detected when his shadow is cast by the sun off to the side of the tree.

Deep shadows are the darker areas created where a solid object blocks the passage of light. A shelter set up in an area of heavy brush may not cast a shadow, but when viewed from a distance may result in a darker area or deeper shadows. Deep shadows are most easily detected from the air.

SHINE

Shine is the reflection of light off any object. Perhaps one of the best examples of shine is light reflected from a mirror. In fact, using a mirror to reflect light is a common method of signaling for help in a survival situation. However, in an evasion scenario you want to avoid shine.

Any reflective object can cause shine, such as the lenses of binoculars, rifle scopes, and flashlights. Bright pieces of metal (such as a knife blade or a metal cup) can also cause shine.

When considering shine, you have to take color into account. Bright colors reflect more light (shine) then darker colors.

SILHOUETTE

A silhouette is any dark shape or outline seen against a light background. A person standing on a hilltop will silhouette himself against the sky. The same effect can occur on a snow field or against the background of a still body of water.

SURFACE

When considering surface, think of size and texture of an object. The greater the surface area of an object, the easier it is to detect. Therefore, when attempting to camouflage something, keep the surface area as small as possible. You can't shrink the physical size of an object, but you can reduce the exposed surface of that object. A man squatting in an open field is more difficult to see than a man standing in the field, all other things being equal. A small camp is more difficult to spot than a large one.

SOUND

A man may be invisible yet give himself away because he is making noise. Sound carries and allows a searcher to detect your location long before he could possibly see you. Detectable sound includes footsteps, conversations, radio noise, gunshots, among others.

Louder and sharper sounds are easier to detect than softer sounds. A gunshot is much easier to hear than a whisper. When attempting to evade detection, it is important to remain quiet or at least to consider the possibility that any sound you make may give you away.

SMELL

Like sound, smell can be detected long before a searcher can see you. Smell may be underrated as a means of detection in our modern society, but it is vitally important to the wilderness evader. The smell of the smoke from a campfire may be detected even if the smoke is not. Cigarette smoke, perfumes, aftershave lotions, and even human body odor can all be detected. It is important to consider the potential of odors being detected when planning your camouflage. This is especially true if dogs are used to search for you.

MOVEMENT

Finally, we come to movement. Movement naturally attracts attention. If you spot a friend across the street you may wave to attract his attention. If two people are standing at the edge of a wood and one begins walking while the other remains still, the moving man will be seen first. If you think that someone may be looking at you, remain still. Lack of movement may cause him to look right past you. If you must move, make your movements slow and smooth. Erratic movements attract attention much more quickly than slow, deliberate movements.

Now that you know the principles of camouflage, you need to consider how to employ them. When assembling your equipment, it is important to consider S7M, but in doing so you also need to ensure that your overall appearance does not make you stand out and become memorable to anyone who might see you. It may be better to avoid camouflage-pattern clothing when simple dark-colored clothing will accomplish much the same thing. Military-style equipment makes you stand out in a nonmilitary environment. Therefore, you should try to limit the use of military gear. Remember that anyone who happens to see you should simply see another backpacker or camper. This overall concept is known as deception and is intended to make the opposition believe that you are other than what you really are.

Chapter 16

Food

Although food is not the first priority in a survival/evasion situation, sooner or later getting something to eat has to be done. A person skilled in woodcraft can live off the land in a friendly environment and probably survive in fairly hostile environments, as well. However, spending all one's time gathering food, trapping, and hunting game is not the best option for the wilderness evader. Even the "mountain men" of the 1800s took provisions with them and made arrangements to resupply themselves at rendezvous and trading posts.

I like to have plenty of food prepared and packaged in my GOOD kit and cached in my planned evasion area. Having basic bulk foods cached allows you to live in an area even if you are unable gather food or hunt and trap game. You can then use the game you catch and the plants you gather to supplement your stored bulk foods.

A cache containing oatmeal, rice, flour, pasta, split peas, nuts, sugar, dried beans, and powdered whole milk can go a long way toward meeting your dietary needs. Supplement this with peanut butter, honey, canned meats, coffee, tea, and other personal favorites, and your meals will come close to normal fare.

BANNOCK

In Scotland bannock is a flat oatmeal and barley cake. However, here in the United States bannock is a survival food that I learned about from Karen Hood at the Hoods Woods survival school in Idaho. Karen has produced a series of videos called "Cave Cooking" (this a companion series to the one produced by her husband, Ron, "Woodsmaster Survival Videos"), that provides excellent instruction for food preparation in remote-area survival. The Hoods have a Web site at <http://www.survival.com>, where you can order the videos and much more.

Bannock is a flour mixture that can be used to make bread, thicken soups, or provide a coating for game and fish caught in the wild. I make bannock and keep a couple of pounds of it in my pack whenever I'm in the backwoods. I've found that it makes an excellent survival food that keeps for at least several weeks after being made if it is stored in a reasonably airtight container. I keep mine rolled up is a couple of plastic bags in my pack.

To make bannock you use the following:

> 1 cup flour
> 1 teaspoon baking powder
> 1/4 teaspoon salt
> 2 tablespoons powdered skim milk
> 3 tablespoons margarine

Sift the dry ingredients together, making sure they are thoroughly mixed. To the dry ingredients, add the margarine and mix until it is completely dispersed throughout the dry ingredients. At this time the mixture should have a consistency similar to granules of sand. The mixture sticks together a little if squeezed between your fingers.

This bannock mixture can be used like flour in your wilderness recipes. For example, add a little water to bannock to make a dough that you can then wrap around a stick and cook over an open fire to make a tasty bread. Bannock is definitely worth considering as an addition to your wilderness food supplies.

TRAPPING

Trapping will be your primary means of obtaining meat for your diet. Properly set traps work for you when you are doing other things and even while you are sleeping. Any animal can be trapped, but our focus is usually on small game, such as squirrels and rabbits. Less commonly eaten animals, such as raccoons and opossums, can also be trapped and eaten—and when properly prepared really don't taste too bad.

Conibear Traps

I recommend that you cache a number of traps in your planned survival area and that you have two or three traps in your GOOD kit. The Conibear trap, invented by and named for Frank Conibear around 1958, is my recommendation for trapping in a survival situation. The Conibear trap is a body-gripping trap, designed to kill the animal. It is basically two metal rods formed into squares, hinged at their center, and designed to spin around their centerpoint by spring tension when the trigger is released.

Conibear traps come in various sizes, but the three most popular sizes are 110, 220, and 330. The 110 trap measures 4 1/2 inches square and is used to catch squirrels, rabbits, pheasants, and possibly fish. The 220 measures 7 inches square and is useful for catching raccoons, geese, skunks, and other animals of similar size. The 330 is designed for trapping beaver but could also be used to catch other animals in the 30-pound range. For survival purposes, I like the 110 and maybe a couple of 220 traps. Unless I was specifically planning to trap beaver I would pass on the 330 Conibear because it is too big for most survival trapping.

Snares

In addition to Conibear traps, snares are an essential part of your survival trapping gear. A snare is simply a piece of wire or cord with a slip-loop on one end that is set in such a way to tighten around any animal passing through it. For small game you can use 16- to 20-gauge stainless-steel wire. Larger animals, such as raccoons, tend to fight the snare until they break the wire. For larger animals, you can use steel fishing leader wire to make your own snares or purchase commercial snares. Because survival trapping focuses on small animals, I keep a spool of wire in my kit to make snares. However, because commercial snares are stronger and generally very inexpensive, I keep several of them cached with my other traps.

The simplest snare to set is the drag snare. It is set on a trail along which you expect an animal to pass. You'll see paths where animals run and holes where they've make their dens. Set a snare on these paths, and the next time an animal comes along it will likely push through the snare, which will tighten around it and hold it in place. When setting a drag snare it is often necessary to place sticks on either side of the snare, forming a fence or gate area to direct the animal into the snare.

If there are squirrels in the area, in addition to setting snares on the ground,

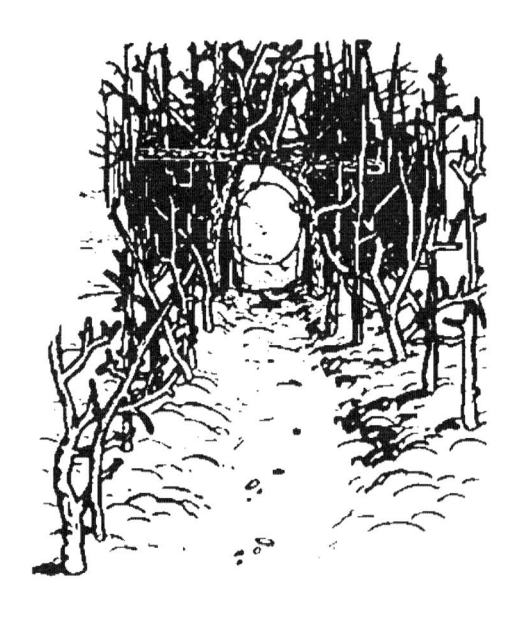

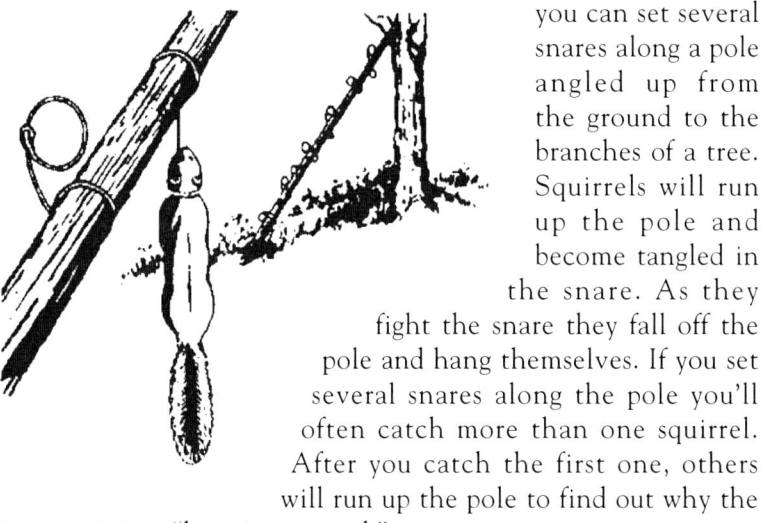

FOOD

you can set several snares along a pole angled up from the ground to the branches of a tree. Squirrels will run up the pole and become tangled in the snare. As they fight the snare they fall off the pole and hang themselves. If you set several snares along the pole you'll often catch more than one squirrel. After you catch the first one, others will run up the pole to find out why the first one is just "hanging around."

Many survival manuals show ways to make snares that lift an animal off of the ground by using a bent sapling or the like. These are commonly called "tip-up snares." Personally, I don't think these traps are useful if you are trying to hide your presence. They take time and effort to construct and tend to stand out much more than a piece of wire along an animal trail. In fact, snares are generally very difficult to see (which is why they catch things), so it is important to make sure you know exactly where you set a snare—or you may not find it again. Tip-up snares with their bent poles, counterweights, and other parts stand out. They also require much more wire or cord to set effectively.

Deadfalls

The deadfall is a crushing trap. It is a weight, such as a log or large rock, supported by a trigger system that when touched causes the weight to fall and crush the prey below it. The deadfall can be designed to kill an animal of almost any size, but for survival trapping it is primarily used for small game.

One advantage of the deadfall is that it can be built from all-natural materials. This construction helps to camouflage the trap; however, anyone seeing the set deadfall will have no difficulty in determining that it is artificial.

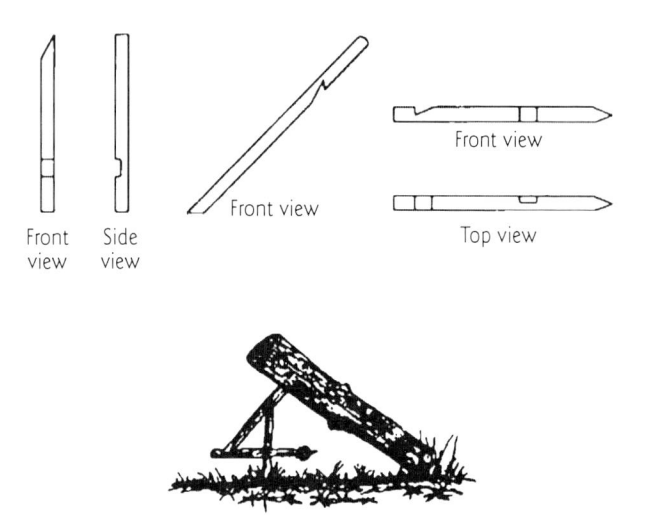

Figure 4 Deadfall

There are several ways to construct a deadfall, but the most common is the figure 4. The figure 4 deadfall is made from three sticks, notched to stay together in a figure "4" pattern when weight is placed on the diagonal stick, but the structure is to fall apart when the horizontal stick is moved.

In some cases the weight of the deadfall won't kill the animal that triggers it. I have found that by placing wooden spikes in the deadfall the animal is both crushed and impaled on the spikes. This helps ensure a clean kill and prevents the possibility of merely wounding an animal.

Paiute Deadfall

A second type of deadfall is the Paiute deadfall, which incorporates a piece of cord into the trigger system, making it a bit more sensitive than that of the figure 4. The cord takes the place of part of the trigger stick. To set the

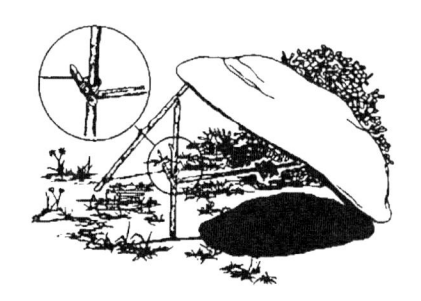

Paiute deadfall, connect a cord to the base of the diagonal stick and a toggle to the other end of the cord. The cord should be just long enough to reach the vertical stick and allow for a one-half turn around it. Now, brace a trigger stick between the toggle and the weight of the deadfall. Moving the trigger stick causes the cord's end to slip off the toggle and the whole thing to fall on whatever disturbed the trigger.

Other Traps

In addition to Conibear traps, snares, and deadfalls, there are other ways to catch animals.

Coffee-Can Trap

Bury a 1-pound coffee can (though it only holds about 13 ounces these days) so that the open top is level with the surface of the earth. Next scatter seeds on the ground around the opening and place more seeds in the bottom of the can. Birds will eat the seeds around the opening and will often jump into the can to get the seeds at its bottom. The small diameter of the can prevents the bird from flapping its wings to fly out, and it will not be able to jump straight up to get out.

Rat Trap

A rat trap is just a big mouse trap. It can be found in most hardware stores and in many grocery stores. When bait is placed on the trigger pan, the rat trap can be used to catch birds, squirrels (which are just furry rats), rabbits, and other small game. Before using rat traps to catch game, it pays to drill a small hole through the wooden base to allow the trap to be fixed in place.

Quail Cup Trap

It is sometimes possible to catch quail by using a paper cup or some birchbark made into a cone. Coat the inside of the cup or the cone with pine pitch or another sticky substance. Place the cup on the ground on its side. Scatter some seeds around the cup, and put some more seeds at the bottom of the cup. A quail feeding on the seeds will push its head into the cup to get the seeds at the bottom.

The pine pitch makes the cup stick over the head of the quail. Now, the quail not being able to see (perhaps thinking the sun has set and it is night) just sits down and goes to sleep. You need only walk up to the quail and grab it.

EDIBLE PLANTS

There is a wide variety of edible wild plants in many wilderness environments. Of course, the specific plants available depend on location and season. I believe that anyone who ventures into the wilderness should be familiar with such plants in his intended area.

Such plants as burdock, cattail, dandelion, pine, and plantain are found pretty much everywhere. Other edible wild plants may be found only in certain regions. I suggest that you learn the edible wild plants found in your area. Actually get out and identify these plants in the field. Gather them and prepare them with your meals. You'll find some that you enjoy, and probably some you dislike, but you'll know what plants can be used for food when necessary. Another advantage of learning to recognize and use edible wild plants is that this provides a supplement to your regular meals.

You may come across a plant that is abundant in your area but that you don't know whether it is edible or not. (Just eating a bunch of it anyway is a pretty bad idea if it turns out to be poisonous.) There is a way to test plants for edibility that lets you safely determine whether you can eat a portion of it.

Universal Edibility Test

To perform the universal edibility test, first make sure that the plant you want to test is abundant in the area you want to retreat to. It makes little sense to go through the effort of performing the test if there is a limited supply of that plant to begin with. Now follow these steps:

- Test each part of the plant separately (e.g., stems, roots, leaves, flowers). Some plants have both edible and inedible parts.
- Smell the plant for strong acid-like odors. Smell

alone won't tell you whether a plant may be eaten safely, but unfamiliar plants with strong odors should be avoided.
- Test the plant for contact poison by rubbing a piece of it in a small area on the inside of your forearm. If the plant is poisonous the skin will generally be affected within a half-hour. (Remember, however, that poison ivy, poison oak, and poison sumac can take days to react. Learn to recognize and avoid these three plants!)
- Take a piece of the plant and touch it to the inside of you lip. See whether this causes any burning or itching within about 5 minutes.
- If touching the plant to your lip caused no burning or itching, hold it in your mouth for about 15 minutes. Do *not* chew it and do *not* swallow.
- If holding it in your mouth caused no burning or itching, chew a piece and hold it in your mouth for another 15 minutes. Do *not* swallow it for those 15 minutes. If no burning or itching occurs, swallow the piece of plant you have been chewing.
- Now wait 8 hours. You should feel no ill effects. If the plant makes you sick, induce vomiting and drink large amounts of water to help flush it from your system.
- Finally, if you had no ill effects from any of the above testing, prepare 1/4 cup of the plant and eat it. Wait another 8 hours. If you feel no ill effects, the plant is safe to eat.

It is important when testing a plant for edibility to prepare it in the manner you want to use it for food. If you plan to eat the plant raw, then test it raw. If you plan to boil it before eating, then perform your edibility test on a boiled plant.

As you can see from the instructions, performing the universal edibility test takes at least 17 hours and only identifies one portion of one plant at a time as being either edible or inedible. For someone planning to be in a wilderness area, it makes sense to learn the edible wild plants in the area and to know how to prepare them. Even if you have no plans for moving to a wilderness area, it still pays to know a few plants that can be safely eaten—after all, things happen!

FISHING

In an area with a body of water (stream, river, pond, lake, ocean) fish can be a pleasant addition to a survivor's diet. Fish are something with which we are all familiar, and they do not take on the connotation of "survival food" in the way that other things may. In some areas fish may be plentiful, and in other area less so, but they are always worth considering as a food source.

The traditional method of sitting on the bank with a fishing pole is a pleasant way to spend an afternoon, but simply isn't an efficient means of fishing for the survivor. To catch fish in a survival/evasion situation what is wanted is a method of catching fish that does not require constant attention and is not easily detected by searchers.

Lets take a look at some of these methods.

Trotline

A trotline is a main line strung in the water with several baited lines coming off the main line. To make a trotline start with a strong main line. I like to use 550 parachute cord, but any type of strong cord will work. Beginning at the center of the main line, tie a secondary line (the baited lines) every 2 feet. The baited lines should be made from 12-pound-test fish line. Tie a hook and sinker to each of the secondary lines. The baited lines should be between 2 and 3 feet long.

Bait each hook with a worm, grub, bug, or whatever you think will likely attract fish. Now stretch the line in the water, tying it between two submerged stakes. If you are fishing for bottom feeders, let the line sink to the bottom. If you are fishing for top feeders, pull the main line tight to lift the baited lines off the bottom. In some cases, it may be possible to tie one end of the trotline to a

FOOD

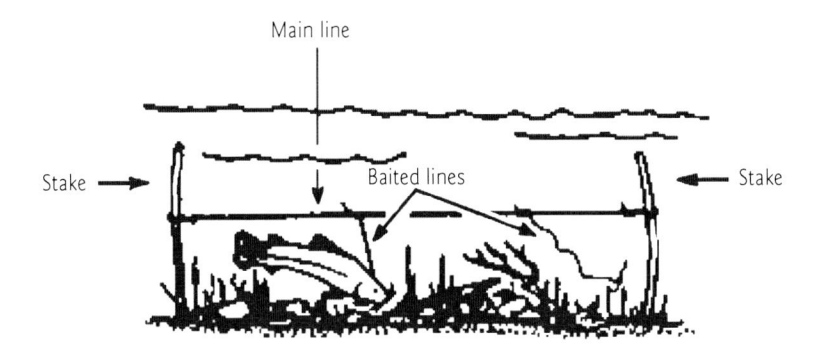

Diagram labels: Main line, Stake, Baited lines, Stake

rock that is cast out into deep water and to tie the other end near the shore. This causes the line to angle down into deep water with some baited lines resting on the bottom while others are suspended higher up. In all cases, however, the entire trotline should be underwater and hidden from view.

Once the trotline is set, you can go about other business, leaving the trotline to do its work. Set the trotline in the morning and then check it around sunset. Gather your fish and reset the line, checking it again in the morning. Depending on the length of your line and the difficulty of the area in which you are setting it, it will probably take about 20 minutes to set the trotline. This will catch quite a few fish yet requires only a few minutes' work on your part each day. Since the trotline is set underwater it is unlikely to be detected by searchers or passersby. However, because it is difficult to see, be sure that you clearly remember where you set it or leave some obscure mark on the bank allowing you to locate it again.

Fish Trap

An excellent method for catching fish is a fish trap. The first time I tried a fish trap it caught fish, and almost every time I used it thereafter it has been successful. Although a fish trap takes a little time to build, it can be used over and over again successfully.

You can think of a fish trap as a basket with a funnel at one end. The fish swim into the trap through the funnel, are are unable to find their way back out. A large fish trap will usually catch a few fish every time it is placed in the water.

To make a fish trap, you need several thin, straight branches or saplings and four or five thicker saplings that can be shaped and bent into hoops. Begin by bending the thicker saplings into hoops with a diameter of 18 to 30 inches. You usually have to whittle these saplings a little to get them to bend in a full circle. Lash the ends together so that you have hoops for your basket. Now lash the thinner saplings around the hoops to form the walls of the basket. These saplings should be lashed onto the hoops so that they have gaps of only about 1/2 inch between them. Once the basket is done, build a funnel that extends into the open end of the basket. The large end of the funnel is the same diameter as the open end of the basket, and the thin end of the funnel should have an opening of around 3 inches.

I found that if the ends of the sticks on the narrow end of the funnel are sharpened the fish are less likely to try swimming back out the opening. I guess they don't like getting poked with a sharp stick. The funnel should be tied into the open end of the basket but should be able to be easily untied and removed to allow you to get fish from the trap. When completed, your fish trap should be about 2 feet in diameter and about 5 feet long. The funnel should extend about 18 inches into the trap.

This may sound like a bit of a construction project, and to be honest it does take a bit of time to build and you do need plenty of cord or wire to lash it all together. However, if you are in a position to come up with some 1/2-inch chicken wire you can construct a fish trap in just a few minutes. Make the basket and funnel from a roll of chicken wire. A piece of chicken wire is cut and securely lashed in place for the bottom of the trap.

To use your fish trap place some bait in the trap. This can be worms or grubs in a mesh bag or perhaps a piece of rotten meat tied on a cord and hung in the center of the trap. Tie the funnel in place and sink your trap in a pond or pool in a stream. You will have to place a couple of rocks in the trap to cause it to sink to the bottom. Now just leave the trap in place, checking it perhaps once per day. If you have taken the time to construct a good, sturdy trap you will catch fish.

Gill Net

A gill net is a great way to catch fish. It is hung in the water and becomes entangled in the fishes' gills as they try to swim through it. It is strung on a line across the top of the net, and the bottom is weighted so that it hangs straight down in the water. As a normal fishing tool, the gill net's top edge is often attached to floats. You shouldn't use the floats because it makes the net (or at least the floats holding it up) highly visible.

To use the gill net, string it between two anchor points, allowing it to hang straight down in the water. The top of the net does not need to be at the surface of the water: in fact, for our purposes it is better to have it a bit underwater to prevent detection. The net can be strung across a stream or in a pond or lake. As long as both ends are anchored and the net hangs straight down in the water, you can use it pretty much anywhere.

Some survival manuals show how to make a gill net using parachute cord or other line. Although this is possible, it's usually much more work than it's worth, and, unless you just happen to have a spare parachute or two, it will cost you more to buy the line to make the net than to buy a commercial gill net. You can buy a 50-by-6-foot gill net for around $25. For survival purposes, I usually cut these nets into two 25-foot lengths because they are easier to handle. You should match the mesh in the net to the size of fish you plan on catching. For survival purposes a 1 1/2-inch mesh is about right. A bunch of smaller fish make as good a meal as a couple of larger fish, and there are always more smaller fish to catch than larger ones.

As with other items that are "set" to catch fish, set your gill net in the morning and check it around sundown. Then collect your fish, reset the net, and check it again the next morning.

An interesting alternative use of a gill net is to string it loosely between a couple of trees to catch birds in flight.

CHAPTER 17

Water

Water is essential to survival. You can live for a few weeks without food, but only a few days without water. Because of this you must ensure that you have a sufficient source of drinking water at all times when you are in the wilderness. Your GOOD kit should contain an initial source of drinking water, but water is heavy and bulky. This means that you'll have to locate other sources of water to replace your initial source. Your two means to provide for long-term water needs are purification and storage systems.

PURIFICATION

Unfortunately, you can't drink just any water you find in the wilderness. Even that crystal-clear, remote mountain stream may be contaminated by the carcass of a dead animal in the water somewhere upstream. The good news is that once you have found a reliable source of water, it is not too difficult to ensure that it is safe for drinking.

The first step in purifying water is to filter out any debris that may be floating in the water you have collected. The filtering process I speak of here is just to remove visible debris in the water and make it more palatable. There is no sense in slurping down a cup of swamp slime if you can filter it out of the water to start with. If the water is clear to begin with, you may choose to skip the filtering process, even though it doesn't hurt to filter it anyway and may improve the taste. Water can be filtered through several layers of cloth, or through alternating layers of sand and charcoal (from your fire). Place layers of sand and charcoal in a container with a small hole in the bottom. Pour water to be filtered into the top of the can and catch the filtered water as it drips out the hole in the bottom of the can.

Now that you have filtered your water you'll need to purify it for drinking. The most effective way of purifying water is to boil it. There are various formulas for how long water should be boiled, but most are not all that important. Just bring the water to a boil and then store it in a clean, covered container. This procedure kills all bacteria in the water and makes it safe for drinking. Most organisms are long dead before the water reaches the boiling point anyway.

It may not always be possible or desirable to boil water. If you're moving rapidly or do not want to risk building a fire, boiling water to purify it is not an option. In this case consider chemical purification. Various chemicals can be used to kill harmful bacteria in the water you intend to drink:

- Bleach (5.25-percent sodium hypochlorite)—3 drops per quart (1 tablespoon per gallon). Note that bleach loses its strength with time, so any bleach you use should be no more than several weeks old.
- Iodine—6 drops per quart, Shake and let stand for 30 minutes before drinking. I prefer Polar Pure Iodine Crystals, but any iodine will work. Note that there is a difference between povidone iodine

solution (Betadine) and pure iodine, but both work well. Iodine has an advantage over bleach in that it can also be used as a topical antiseptic.
- Potassium permanganate—add until water becomes pink in color. Adding more potassium permanganate (until the water becomes a dark pink or red) produces an effective topical antiseptic.

Chemical purification is useful, but it should be noted that it is not 100-percent effective. For example, iodine will not kill cryptosporidium at any concentration you would use in drinking water and is not immediately effective on giardia.

You also have the option of using a microfilter to purify water. This filter consists of a pump unit and a filter system that removes bacteria as well as many chemicals. The Swiss Katadyn filter has a reputation as the best in the world (and it may be), but it's very expensive. I've used other brand-name water filters in many different areas of the world and have never had any problem. Because I use my water filters as a backup means of water purification I use the less expensive models. However, if I had to rely on a filter as a primary purification means, I would go with Katadyn.

One final method of purifying water, recommended by the World Health Organization in certain Third World countries, is to place water in clear containers in strong sunlight for several hours. Based on personal experiments, I can say that this method is somewhat effective, but not 100 percent by any means. I guess that if you are trying to provide drinking water for some African village where the population bathes, drinks, and urinates in the same pool, this method is better than nothing. However, if you are in an area that offers several hours of strong sunlight each day, and you are purifying water for one person or even a few people, you can use a solar oven to boil the water and be sure of killing all harmful organisms.

STORAGE

Disaster preparedness manuals teach that you should store a minimum of 1 gallon of water per person per day. This is good advice, and for the wilderness evader a base camp (and any other semipermanent camps) should have a stored supply of fresh drinking water. If your camp is located near any body of water (e.g., stream, spring, pond), you have a good source of water, but you won't want to take time to purify it each time you want a glass of water. Thus, you need to provide a container to store water at your camp. This is generally not a problem; simply set up a water storage container at your base camp and keep it filled with treated water when you are there. I found a 15-gallon collapsible water bag at a military surplus store that works well for me. I keep it cached near my camp and fill it on my arrival and refill it as I drink from it.

CHAPTER **18**

Survival Medicine

WARNING: The advice in this chapter is not intended to replace care and treatment by medical professionals when they are available to provide care and treatment. Survival medicine assumes that you do not have access to a physician or medical facility but still must treat personal illness or injury. While you learn survival medicine, I recommend that you focus on your individual health and circumstances and that you consult your personal physician for additional advice.

Illness and injuries are foremost among the problems that can seriously compromise your ability to remain in a wilderness environment and evade detection by others. What might be a mere inconvenience in a more populated environment, with prompt access to medical attention, can quickly become life-threatening without medical attention. A sprained ankle at home may mean a couple of weeks of hobbling around on crutches; in the wilderness it may restrict your movements so as to make evasion difficult, if not impossible. A bad case of the flu at home may mean a few days in bed; in the wilderness if you are unable to hole up and rest, it can be a killer.

In addition there are illnesses and injuries that are more commonly associated with wilderness environments. Cold-induced injuries (e.g., frostbite, hypothermia) and heat-induced injuries (e.g., heat cramps, heatstroke) are commonly considered "outdoor injuries." Insect bites from mosquitoes, ticks, and wasps are also generally a problem of much more concern to someone in the outdoors.

MEDICAL TRAINING

Survival medicine is much more than just first aid. For our purposes, survival medicine is defined as "definitive treatment of illnesses and injuries that does not depend on the availability of technical medical assistance." In other words, survival medicine is do-it-yourself medicine. This does not mean, however, that survival medicine is administered without some degree of training and forethought. In fact, the greater your medical knowledge, the better your treatment.

To obtain some proficiency in survival medicine you must begin your training somewhere. Unlike most writers who discuss survival medicine, I do not recommend the Red Cross first-aid course. The Red Cross is a fine organization, but its course is far too basic—and has come to cost too much since the Red Cross started charging for the course—to be of much value for our purposes. You can learn as much, if not more, about basic first aid by studying the books in the survival medicine section of the bibliography of this book. Also, take a look at Dr. Richard Harvey's comments in the February 2001 issue of *Nine-One-One News*. Harvey discusses a study from the Harvard School of Education, where two groups of individuals were taught cardiopulmonary resuscitation (CPR). One group took the standard 4-hour course, while the second group was shown a half-hour video and then practiced on a mannequin. The groups were then tested to see how they performed CPR. *The video group outperformed the standard-course group by a wide margin.* Unless you have absolutely no clue about basic

SURVIVAL MEDICINE

first aid, begin your training with self-study and then move on to more advanced training.

To get more advanced medical training I recommend that you take an emergency medical technician (EMT) course. Many community colleges offer the basic EMT course, which is based on standards established by the U.S. Department of Transportation. An EMT course gives you a minimum of 110 hours of instruction, including practical hands-on training and "live environment" training (you will be required to complete a shift in a hospital emergency room). Once you've completed the EMT training (and passed the state's certification exam), you can probably volunteer with your local fire, medical, or ambulance service, as well as back at the hospital where you did your initial training. This gives you a way of maintaining and updating your skills, as well as regular contacts with doctors, nurses, and other medical personnel who may be willing to teach you additional medical techniques useful in a wilderness environment.

Depending on where you live and the depth of your interest in survival medicine, you may want to attend courses that specialize in wilderness medicine. There are many such courses available, but if you aren't aware of a course in your area you can contact one of the following organizations for more information.

Wilderness Medical Associates
189 Dudley Road
Bryant Pond, ME 04219

SOLO Wilderness Emergency Medicine
P.O. Box 3150
Conway, NH 03818

Wilderness Medicine Institute, Inc.
413 Main Street
P.O. Box 9
Pitkin, CO 81241

Let's look now at some of the basics of survival medicine that everyone should know, regardless of what other training you may have.

PERSONAL HYGIENE

The most important part of survival medicine is personal hygiene. If you are not sick or injured, good hygiene helps prevent illness. If you are sick or injured, good hygiene speeds recovery.

Washing is the best way to prevent the spread of germs and helps to prevent small scrapes, scratches, and abrasions (common in the wilderness) from becoming infected. At least you should wash your hands, face, and feet every day. A complete sponge bath is better, and of course a hot shower is ideal. Water can be heated over a fire with little effort. On occasion it may be possible to visit campgrounds that have shower facilities, and if you are in an area where leaving signs of your presence is not a concern, showers or saunas may be easily improvised.

If water is not available or is in short supply you can still take an "air bath." Remove all clothing and simply expose your body to the air and sun. Shake out your clothing and hang it in the open air. Just be careful while you have your backside basking in the sun to avoid sunburn.

Comb your hair daily and wash it regularly. This prevents parasites from making themselves at home in your tresses. A comb should be included in your GOOD kit. If for some reason you have lost your comb, it is possible to carve one from a piece of wood, although this takes longer than you might expect.

In addition to the hygienic advantages of keeping your hair clean and combed, a clean appearance makes you less memorable to anyone who might happen to see you. With a reasonably neat appearance you may be accepted as just another hiker. On the other hand, if you are so grubby and matted that you look like Big Foot's cousin, you will be remembered. Along the same line, a razor and a pair of scissors to stay clean-shaven or to maintain a trimmed beard has the same advantages as keeping your hair clean and combed.

SURVIVAL MEDICINE

Oral Care

Another very important aspect of personal hygiene in a wilderness environment is oral care. A toothache probably isn't a life-threatening injury, but it may make you wish you would die. It will certainly distract you from other matters. A toothbrush takes up very little space and should definitely be included in the items you carry with you into the wilderness.

If you don't have a toothbrush you can make a "chew stick" to help keep your teeth clean. Get a clean stick and chew one end until it is frayed and brushlike. The frayed end can be used to clean your teeth. Whittle a point on the other end to use as a toothpick. A clean piece of cloth can be wrapped around the end of a stick to make a toothbrush. And if nothing else is available simply rubbing your teeth and gums with your finger helps remove food particles. You can even make a mouthwash by steeping willow bark in hot water to make a tea. Gargling with willow bark tea helps protect your teeth and gums.

Oral bleeding, such as from a lost tooth, can be controlled by using a tea bag as a compress. The tannic acid in the tea is a vasoconstrictor that helps to stop the bleeding and, perhaps, reduce the pain.

Foot Care

Care of your feet in a survival situation is of the utmost importance. Your feet may be your only means of transportation, and if you have difficulty walking you certainly won't be able to evade effectively.

To care for your feet, you should wash and dry them daily. If you have foot powder, you should use it. Keep your toenails trimmed straight across to prevent ingrown toenails. Examine your feet regularly for red spots or blisters and cover these areas with moleskin or adhesive tape.

Make sure that your boots are well broken in but not worn out before wearing them into the wilderness. Socks should fit well, and not be so large that they get wrinkled, which can cause blisters. Wool socks are probably the best material for use in the wilderness. However, some people don't like the feel of wool against their skin. In this case a thin pair of cotton socks can be worn as an inner layer and the wool socks worn over the cotton pair. Keep socks as clean and dry as possible and carry fresh socks in your GOOD kit.

Clothing and Bedding

As important as keeping your body clean is keeping clean the clothing you wear and the bedding you sleep in. As clothing becomes dirty it should be washed. Admittedly, in a wilderness area this isn't as simple as dropping clothing off at the local dry cleaners, but you still should make every attempt to keep your clothing clean.

When you are camped in an area for a day or more, you can wash dirty items and hang them in the sun to dry. At a minimum, clothing should be shaken out and hung in the air for as many hours as possible.

Bedding should be shaken out and hung up to air daily. When possible, bedding should be washed regularly and hung in the sun to dry. Cleaning blankets and sleeping bags is a bit more difficult than washing clothing, but it is still necessary to clean bedding from time to time to prevent disease.

REST

In addition to personal hygiene, it is essential that one gets enough rest to maintain good health. Rest restores physical energy, clears thinking, and promotes healing of injuries and illnesses. The amount of rest a person needs depends on his health, the amount of work he does (and thus the amount of energy burned up) and his individual makeup.

Traditionally, a person is supposed to get 8 hours of sleep a night, but in actuality one may need as little as 4 or 5 hours or as much as 10 or 12 hours. The point is that you should maintain a schedule of sleep time every day. Too often in survival situations people work themselves to exhaustion, collapse for a few hours, and then work themselves to exhaustion again. This quickly breaks down health. If it's at all possible, even in a survival situation, plan to give yourself 6 or 8 hours sleep each night.

In addition to proper sleep each night, you should schedule breaks throughout the day. The amount of time and the number of breaks needed depends on the type and amount of work you are doing, but an average of approximately 10 minutes per hour is generally about right.

INJURY MANAGEMENT

We will not go over the basics of first aid here: this topic is covered extensively in the books listed in the survival medicine section of the bibliography. Furthermore, if you have completed EMT training, you already know much more than basic first aid. However, we will look at some wilderness-related injuries as they apply to the survivor and evader.

Thorns and Splinters

Thorns and splinters are fairly common when working in a wilderness environment. If properly treated these injuries are not usually a serious problem. The first step you want to take regarding thorns and splinters is to prevent getting injured by them in the first place by wearing proper gloves and boots. If you do get stuck with a thorn or splinter, make sure that you remove it quickly and completely. It is important to make sure you remove all pieces of the thorn or splinter to prevent the wound's becoming infected. Then wash and disinfect the wound and keep it clean. Cover the area with a clean dressing and bandage.

Poisonous Plants
(Poison Ivy, Oak, and Sumac)

Poison ivy, poison oak, and poison sumac all contain a resin that can cause severe skin irritation. The resin is active in all parts of the plant at all times of the year. The plants' effect varies from person to person and may be different at each exposure.

Skin irritation from contact with any of these plants may develop within a couple of hours or may be delayed for several days. The irritation takes the form of red patches or streaks, followed by blisters that later break and result in crusting and oozing from the rash. All of this is generally accompanied by itching, which is often quite severe.

Poison ivy

Poison oak

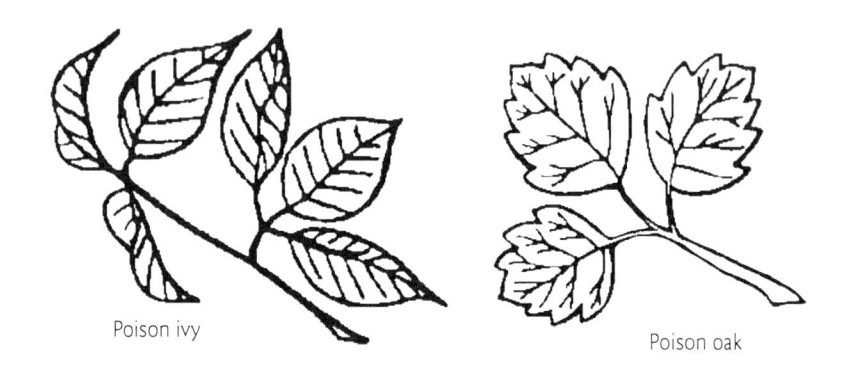

Poison sumac

Treatment following contact with any of these plants includes washing to remove any additional resin from the skin or in the clothes. Cold, wet compresses made from saltwater may provide some relief from the itching. It is important to avoid scratching the rash because this may lead to infection. Scratching the rash, however, will not result in its spreading, as is sometimes asserted, because the fluid in the blisters is not the plant resin that causes the rash itself. The rash usually fades after about a week. Some people have had success in preventing and treating the effects of poison ivy and poison oak by using the crushed leaves of the jewel weed plant. Jewel weed tends to grow in the same areas as both poison ivy and poison oak.

Both poison ivy and poison oak leaves grow in clusters of three. Poison sumac has a varying number of leaves. It is useful for anyone who spends any time in the wilderness to learn to recognize and avoid these plants.

Blisters and Abrasions

Blisters and abrasions are another common wilderness injury, especially for people who are not used to living and working in a wilderness environment. Blisters on the feet can be quite severe, preventing you from hiking, and if the blisters become infected this only compounds the problem. Likewise, blisters may develop on your hands if you engage in heavy physical labor that you are not used to. Again gloves and proper-fitting socks and boots can help prevent blisters. If you do get a blister do not remove the top layer of skin. Doing so only opens the blister area to infection. The best treatment for blisters in a survival situation is to wash and dry the area and cover it with a clean dressing, moleskin, or adhesive tape.

Insect Bites and Stings

Insects can be a major problem for the wilderness survivor and evader. Mosquitoes, flies, wasps, ticks, and chiggers can cause infections from scratched bites as well as transmit various diseases, such as Rocky Mountain spotted fever. Insect repellent is essential in some areas and useful in most others. You should not scratch insect bites. Inspect your body regularly for ticks. If you find any, remove them by pulling them off using tweezers. You should not use heat to remove the tick because this increases the likelihood that contamination will enter the bite wound. Applying a cold, wet cloth to any insect bite areas helps reduce itching and swelling.

Snakebite

The chances of being bitten by a snake in the wilderness are pretty slim. Snakes tend to avoid humans and will leave given half a chance. Furthermore, if you do see a snake, the chances are good that it is not poisonous. In the United States, we have to concern ourselves with just four poisonous snakes: rattlesnakes, cottonmouths, copperheads, and coral snakes. The first three types of snakes are pit vipers, while the coral snake is an elapid. Although the bite of anyone of these snakes can, and has, caused fatalities, the chances of actually dying from the bite of a poisonous snake is about 1 in 12 million. In the case of rattlesnakes and cottonmouths, 20 to 30 percent of bites do not inject venom anyway. In

Pit Vipers

Labels: Fangs, Teeth, Poison sac, Fangs, Poison sac, Fang marks, Teeth marks, Eye, Eye

Coral snake

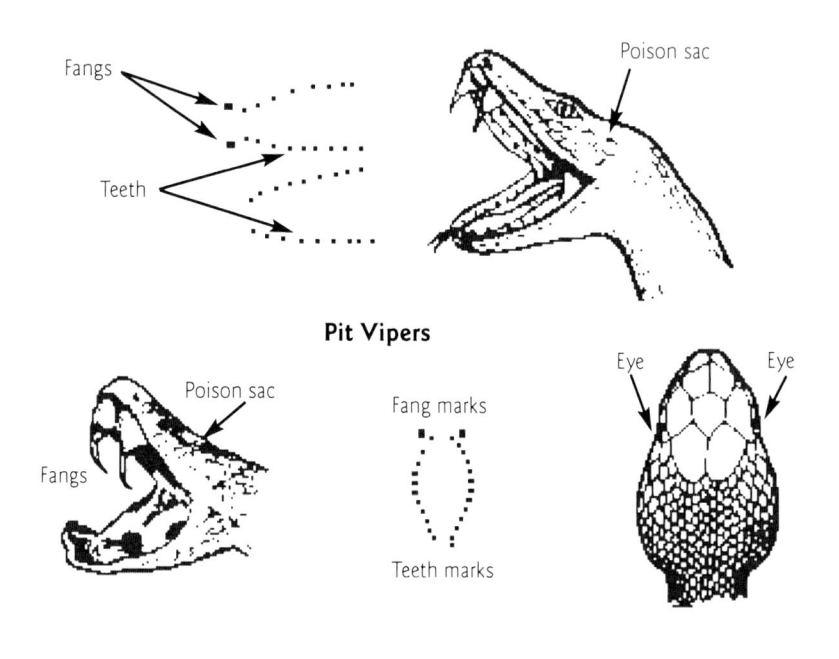

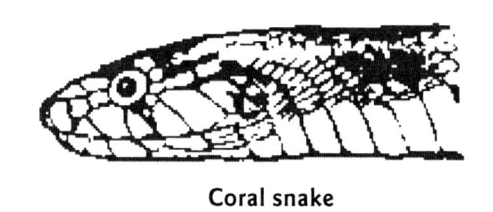

the case of the coral snake, it injects its venom by chewing only, so rapid withdrawal of the very small extremity that it can grab onto may prevent a poisonous bite.

The above having been said, it is important to treat any snakebite as a serious injury. The bite should be treated by keeping the victim calm. Remove any rings or other jewelry because a bitten extremity may swell. Apply a constricting band above and below the bite site. This is *not* a tourniquet and should not stop blood flow. The constricting band is intended only to slow the spread of venom. You should be able to slide a finger between the constricting band and the injured extremity.

SURVIVAL MEDICINE

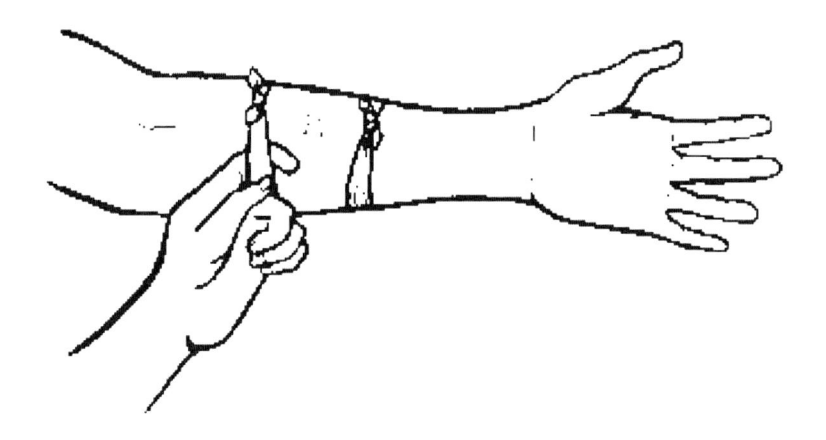

If you have a Sawyer extraction device available, use it. This device *used immediately* can extract about one-third of the injected poison. Wash the bite area with soap and water. Immobilize the bitten area (splint and sling), but keep the wound below the level of the heart. Treat the patient for shock.

There are also a lot of myths about proper treatment of snakebite. Some things not to do are these:

- DO NOT make cuts over the bite marks.
- DO NOT suck the venom out with your mouth.
- DO NOT put ice on the bite.
- DO NOT use rubber bulbs or suction cups – they are ineffective.
- DO NOT apply a tourniquet.
- DO NOT use electrical shock.
- DO NOT consume alcohol.
- DO NOT take aspirin, which increases bleeding.

Cold-Related Injuries

Hypothermia

Hypothermia is the lowering of the body's core temperature. Everybody is familiar with the fact that normal body temperature is around 98.6 degrees Fahrenheit. As the body temperature begins to sink below its normal range, a state of mild hypothermia is reached at around 95 degrees. At this point there are shivering, some lack of coordination, slowed pace, and perhaps mild confusion.

As the body temperature continues its decrease, there are severe lack of coordination and uncontrollable shivering. The individual will likely be stumbling and unable to perform fine motor tasks. Mental sluggishness and moderate confusion is likely present. This occurs with a body temperature around 90 degrees.

As the body temperature falls below 90 degrees, there are a cessation of shivering, an almost complete lack of coordination, and mental incoherence. This is severe hypothermia. Here the body enters a downward spiral into unconsciousness, muscle rigidity, and eventually death from heart failure.

Hypothermia can occur at any air temperature below 82 degrees Fahrenheit but is most common when the temperature is in the 50s. Around this temperature people tend to be "comfortably cool" and do not take the precautions that would be normal in really cold weather. It is essential that hypothermia be treated in its earliest stages. When you feel cold and are shivering, you must stop and get warm. This may be as simple a putting on a hat and sweater or lighting a fire and getting yourself something warm to eat (such as hot soup).

As hypothermia becomes more severe correcting the problem becomes much more difficult. It is essential to get into shelter and wrap up in blankets or a sleeping bag to prevent further cooling. At this state the warm cup of soup simply won't do it. Sugar is also needed to help the body generate its own heat: drinking warm sugar water can help here, as will boiling water and inhaling the steam. The intent here is to immediately stop further cooling and rewarm the body's core.

Frostbite

Frostbite is the freezing of the skin. It can occur even when the temperature is not all that cold, because there is the chilling effect of the wind. Hands, feet, face, and ears are the areas of the body most likely to get frostbite because they are most commonly exposed to the environment.

Frostbite is treated by rapid rewarming of the affected part in warm water at about 104 degrees. Rewarming is only done once the patient has been removed from the cold environment. This thawing of frozen tissue is extremely painful so if pain medicine is available it should be administered to the patient before beginning the rewarming. Care should be taken not to allow the water to be so hot that it causes a burn. Burns are also a possibility when rewarming near a fire or other heat source, so extra caution must be taken to prevent this.

There are some things that should not be done to treat frostbite.

- DO NOT rub the area with snow. This does nothing to re-warm the frozen part and will in fact cause additional damage.
- DO NOT allow the re-warmed part to refreeze.
- DO NOT massage or rub the frozen part of the body.
- DO NOT consume alcohol or use tobacco products when suffering from frostbite.

Heat Injuries

Heat injuries are heat cramps, heat exhaustion, and heat stroke. These injuries tend to be progressive, although a person may be suffering from heat stroke by the time medical treatment is sought.

Cramps

Heat cramps are painful spasms of the muscles from exertion and overheating. Prevention and treatment consist of drinking plenty of water and maintaining salt in the diet. Normally the salt contained in food is sufficient; however, in very hot environments, especially if you must perform heavy labor, an increase of salt may be needed.

Exhaustion

Heat exhaustion, the most common form of heat injury, results from overheating. Signs and symptoms include headache, weakness, nausea and vomiting, and profuse sweating. Treatment consists of getting into a cool (shaded) area, removing restrictive clothing, and drinking cool water. Oral rehydration solutions (e.g., sports drinks) may also be drunk if available to replace electrolytes.

Stroke

Heat stroke is the most serious heat injury. It is a real medical emergency and potentially fatal. Signs and symptoms of heat stroke include high body temperature (105 degrees Fahrenheit or higher), rapid pulse and respiration with a low blood pressure, and often an altered mental status. Sweating may or may not be present. The traditionally described condition of "hot, dry skin" occurs late in the progression and can be misleading: the patient may still be sweating during the early stages of heat stroke. Treatment consists of cooling the patient as quickly as possible (immerse in cool water or pour water over him) and treating for shock. If possible the patient should be evacuated to a medical facility.

Burns

Burns are a possibility in a wilderness environment because of the use of open flames, such as those generated by campfires and stoves. Burns are divided into three categories: superficial (first-degree), partial thickness (second degree), and full thickness (third degree).

Superficial burns are red and painful but are not blistered. Examples of a superficial burn are sunburn and burns from a spilled hot drink. Treatment consists of cooling the area, if possible applying aloe vera gel, and taking ibuprofen (e.g., Motrin or Nuprin) to reduce pain. Although painful, these burns are generally not serious.

Partial-thickness burns are painful, red, and blistered. Treatment consists of cooling the area and removing any dirt or debris that may cause infection. If antibacterial ointment is available, apply it and cover the burn with a dry, nonadhesive, sterile dressing. Ointments and salves that are not antibacterial and not specifically designed for use on burns should not be used because they tend to increase the chance of infection.

Full-thickness burns include all layers of the skin, including the blood vessels, the nerves, and perhaps the muscle tissue. The burn appears dry, charred, and leathery. Because the nerves have been destroyed, full-thickness burns are generally not painful and are often insensitive to touch (areas around the full-thickness burn may have suffered only partial-thickness burns and may be very painful). Full thickness burns constitute a medical emergency, requiring treatment that cannot be effectively given outside a hospital. Treatment consists of covering the burn with dry, sterile, nonadhesive dressing and taking the patient to a hospital. Even under the best conditions full-thickness burns tend to become infected, so hospital care is a must.

With any burn the body suffers a fluid loss. It is important to replace that fluid. If you get burned, it is essential to increase your intake of fluids. This is especially important with partial and full-thickness burns, but should not be overlooked when treating such superficial burns as sunburn.

Pain

Pain from any injury can be a major problem for the survivor. It increases the possibility that he will go into shock, and it makes it much more difficult to concentrate on matters essential to survival and evasion.

Cleaning, bandaging, and splinting (if necessary) the injured area may reduce pain from injuries. Applying heat or cold to the site of the injury may also help reduce pain. Whether to use heat or cold depends on the injury and what makes it feel better for you. Generally, heat may be said to help reduce the pain of a toothache, but you would use cold to help relieve the pain of a sprained ankle.

You should carry aspirin with you. Aspirin is a mild analgesic useful for reducing pain and fever. In the United States all aspirin is the same, so buy the generic brand and save money. It should be noted that ingesting large amounts of aspirin might cause stomach irritation. Furthermore, aspirin should not be given to children as it has been associated with Reye's Syndrome, a postviral encephalopathy and liver failure.

Acetaminophen (i.e., Tylenol) has the same effect as aspirin in relieving pain and reducing fever but has the added benefit of causing less stomach irritation. Ibuprofen (e.g., Motrin) is an anti-inflammatory most commonly used as a mild analgesic. Ibuprofen may be carried in addition to aspirin or acetaminophen to aid in fighting pain.

If you don't have aspirin, you can use willow bark to relieve pain. Willow bark contains salicin, which decomposes into salicyclic acid in the human body. Salicyclic acid is the basis of aspirin. Willow bark may be either chewed (which tastes pretty bad) or made into a tea (which doesn't taste much better) as a means of relieving pain.

To be really effective in controlling pain, you need stronger drugs, such as codeine. However, codeine and other strong painkillers are controlled substances in the United States, and thus you must have a prescription to obtain them.

Shock

Shock is a life-threatening condition and to some extent accompanies all injuries. In many cases shock is more serious than the injury itself. In a wilderness environment you should treat for shock when you suffer any injury. The standard treatment for this is to lie down, keep warm , and elevate the lower extremities to direct blood back to the body's central core.

Psychogenic shock is the body's reaction to extreme stress in a survival situation. The extent to which you are affected by psychogenic shock depends a great deal on your self-confidence and level of training. The treatment for this type of shock is much the same as for any other type of shock, with the intent of the treatment being to allow you to rest, calm yourself, and formulate a plan of action.

The general rule in emergency medicine is that the patient is given nothing to eat or drink before being taken to the hospital. In cases where transport to a hospital is immediate this is of course the correct action. In survival medicine, however, the situation is different: there may be no way to transport you to a hospital. In this case it may be appropriate to drink small amounts of warm liquids (broth or even warm water) if you are conscious, able to swallow, and have no suspected internal injuries. You should, however, never consider ingesting alcohol.

WILDERNESS ILLNESSES

Certain illnesses are associated with a move to a remote or wilderness area. These are almost always the result of making a transition from one environment to another. One living in a remote area tends to be affected less often with the common colds, flus, and viruses found in a heavily populated area.

Diarrhea

Diarrhea is one of the most common illnesses that affect people who move to a wilderness environment. It is often caused by making changes in diet, drinking contaminated water, eating spoiled food, and handling the stress of a survival situation. Diarrhea may be treated by limiting your intake to only liquids for 24 hours. If this does not have the desired effect, an effective antidiarrhea medicine may be made by boiling the bark of hardwoods in water to leach out the tannic acid in the bark. (Acorns can also be boiled to remove the tannic acid and then saved for food.) Boil the bark or acorns for 2 or more hours and then let the solution cool. It will smell bad and taste worse but will generally stop diarrhea. You should drink the solution by the cupful every two hours and drink an additional cup of solution following each bowel movement until the diarrhea stops.

Dehydration

Dehydration is the result of insufficient fluid reserves in the body. Simply put, if you are not drinking enough water, juice, or other liquids to replace fluids lost through the body's natural processes of urination, expiration, and perspiration you become dehydrated.

The average adult loses between 1 and 2 quarts of fluid daily through normal bodily functions. In environments of extreme temperature and at high altitude this fluid loss increases significantly. Add to this the stress of a survival situation and possible injury or illness, and maintaining fluid balance becomes even more important.

The kidneys are very sensitive to the body's fluid levels and react quickly to conserve fluid when there is a reduced intake. When the kidneys are conserving fluids by reducing urination, it is a sign that you may not be drinking enough to replace normal fluid loss.

Urination of less 1/2 quart in a 24-hour period is a sign of dehydration. Urine with a dark color or a strong odor also indicates that you are not drinking sufficient water to replace fluids in your body. When you are consuming enough water your urine should be light in color and without a strong odor. You should also pass about 1 quart of urine every 24 hours.

Other indications of dehydration are thirst, fatigue, dark sunken eyes, emotional instability, loss of skin elasticity, and a trench-like line down the center of the tongue.

To treat dehydration you must replace lost body fluids. This, of course, means drinking water (at least 2 quarts per day). However, since water contains no electrolytes, you should also drink juices, soups, and the like. Avoid coffee and tea; they are diuretics and cause renal fluid loss. You should prevent dehydration by drinking water regularly throughout the day, thus replacing fluid as it is lost. In a very hot environment, you may want to add 1/4 teaspoon of salt to 1 quart of water consumed each day. If you have quite a bit salt in your diet, this may not be necessary, but you should keep it in mind if you are not used to the hot environment or are working at an increased level.

Intestinal Parasites

Intestinal parasites are another illness that can affect the health of a wilderness survivor. Intestinal parasites result from eating undercooked meat or vegetables contaminated with feces. Normally, special medication is required to treat an intestinal parasite infestation in the body, but you may not have these available to you in the wilderness. Expedient methods of killing intestinal parasites rely on changing the environment in the gastrointestinal tract and are not without their own dangers. If you have no other means available, you may use the following remedies to kill intestinal parasites:

- Mix 4 tablespoons of salt in 1 quart of warm water and drink. DO NOT repeat this treatment.

- Eat one or one and a half cigarettes. The nicotine kills the parasites, allowing your system to pass them. This treatment may be repeated in 48 hours if necessary.
- Drink 2 tablespoons of kerosene. Repeat in 48 hours if necessary.

Food Poisoning

Food poisoning is a common threat to the survivor. Food may be improperly preserved and stored, allowing for the development of harmful bacteria. Food poisoning due to performed toxin (staphylococcus or botulism) results in the onset of acute symptoms (nausea, vomiting, and diarrhea) soon after ingesting contaminated food. Resting and consuming large quantities of clean water to flush the system are indicated in this case. If the poisoning is due to ingesting bacteria—determined by the gradual onset of nausea, vomiting, and diarrhea—you should take antibiotics if you have them available. Eating small amounts of fine, clean charcoal can also help relieve the symptoms of food poisoning.

Rashes and Fungal Infections

Rashes and fungal infections are seldom life-threatening problems, but they are uncomfortable and should be treated. The best treatment is to keep an affected area clean and dry. Do not apply alcohol or iodine in an attempt to "burn out" the rash or infection, because this is not effective. Exposing the area to sunlight, however, does help to clear up the problem.

General Treatment

The human body is remarkable in its ability to fight illness and repair itself. In something like 80 percent of the cases where people seek medical treatment they would recover fully from their illnesses or injuries without a physician. Of course the other 20 percent are traumatic injuries and serious illnesses that are too severe for the body to correct. By focusing on general treatment, we can help the body repair itself.

Infection

Infection is a serious threat to someone in a wilderness environment or remote area. Generally, you will not have a large supply of antibiotics to aid in fighting infection. Treatment of infection in a wilderness area must be focused on prevention.

All wounds should be cleaned thoroughly with soap and warm water to help prevent infection. In some cases it may be better to irrigate the wound with a stream of water instead of scrubbing it to limit further tissue damage. Water sprayed in a pressurized stream into a wound can wash out debris and dirt that can lead to infection. A plastic bottle with a small hole drilled in the cap, a plastic bag with the tip of a corner cut off, or a bulb-syringe can all be used to irrigate a wound. *It is essential that the water used to clean a wound be sterile.* It does little good to wash a wound with dirty water. Water boiled for at least 10 minutes and stored in a clean container will remain sterile.

Once the wound has been cleaned, it should be covered with a dry sterile dressing and bandaged to keep dirt and debris from getting back into the wound. The dressings should be changed as necessary and the wound kept clean. If you have antibiotics you should use them. Lacking antibiotics, you can use various natural remedies to help prevent infection. As an example, both the barks of the sweet gum and the American mountain ash have antiseptic properties and can be boiled to make an antiseptic solution for treating wounds.

It is important to remember that even though all wounds need to be cleaned of dirt and debris, antiseptics are best used for cuts, scrapes, abrasions, and small lacerations. External antiseptics applied to large, deep wounds may cause additional tissue damage.

Soaking the wounded area in lukewarm saltwater also helps to draw out the infection. The heat and salt promote oozing of pus from the wound, thereby removing toxins from the wound area.

HERBAL MEDICINE

Almost all our modern medicines have their basis in herbal and natural medicines. Although advances in medicine have certainly developed better treatments and more rapid cures of disease, we don't want to overlook home remedies and the "old country doctor" type of medicine. Particularly with regard to survival medicine, these methods should be studied. In fact, many of the natural remedies are just as effective as the more costly "modern medicine." In with this line, however, it is important to remember that herbal medicines can be misused and that such misuse can be just as harmful as an overdose of any modern drug, so take time to carefully study anything you intend to use as a natural medicine.

It is possible to buy herbal medical kits from many sources. A good basic kit, available from Adventure Medical Kits, contains echinacea, goldenseal extract, ginger extract, arniflora, aloe vera gel, tea tree oil, blister kit items, wound care items, and more. These kits make a good foundation for your herbal medicine inventory, but it is more important to learn what plants are available in your planned evasion area and how to prepared them for use as a medicine (e.g., willow bark as a pain reliever or pine needle tea for vitamin C). Along with this, learn what items you may be carrying for other reasons that also have medical uses (e.g., super glue can be used to treat blisters and lacerations, and cayenne pepper can be used to control bleeding).

COLLOIDAL SILVER

In his excellent article, "A Closer Look at Colloidal Silver," Peter A. Lindemann wrote:

> Colloidal silver is an extraordinary product. It can enhance your health and the health of your family in hundreds of ways. Everyone should learn how to make high quality colloidal silver and have that capability in their home, in case the regulators restrict its availability at some point in the future. This could be the best "health insurance" policy you ever implemented!

But just what is colloidal silver? A colloid is a substance made up of very small, insoluble, indiffusible particles suspended in a liquid. The particles are larger than molecules but small enough so that they cannot easily be filtered and remain suspended in the liquid without settling to the bottom.

Colloidal silver is made by running a low-voltage current through pure silver wire held in distilled water. This results in microscopic particles of silver becoming suspended in the water, forming a colloid.

Silver has always been accepted as treatment for bacteria, virus, and fungal infections. Even today silver compounds are used in the treatment of burns. From the 1920s through the 1940s silver colloids were commonly used as a treatment for many infections and diseases. In 1938 more than 650 bacterial, viral, and fungal infections were considered treatable with colloidal silver.

In the 1996 *Federal Register*, vol. 61, no. 200, pp. 53,685–53,688 we read:

> Colloidal silver is a suspension of silver particles in a colloidal base. Historically, a number of colloidal silver/silver colloidal salts have been marketed in the United States. Some of these colloidal silver products were recognized as official articles in the United States Pharmacopeia (U.S.P.) and the National Formulary (N.F.). Colloidal silver iodide contained not less than 18 percent and not more than 22 percent silver, with the product diluted for local use to concentrations from 0.05 to 10 percent. Strong silver protein (Ref. 1) contained not less than 7.5 percent and not more than 8.5 percent silver, with the product diluted for local use to concentrations from 0.5 to 10 percent. The 10th edition of the N.F. had a cautionary note for these products that stated: "Caution: Solutions of Colloidal Silver Iodide should be freshly prepared and should be dispensed in amber-colored bottles," and "Caution: Strong Silver Protein Solutions should be freshly prepared and should be dispensed in amber-colored bottles." Mild silver protein contained not less than 19 percent and not more than 23 percent silver, with the product diluted for local use to concentrations from 0.1 to 5 percent. The 12th edition of the

N.F. had a cautionary note, which stated: "Caution: Solutions of Mild Silver Protein should be freshly prepared or contain a suitable stabilizer, and should be dispensed in amber-colored bottles."

As pharmaceutical laboratories began to develop and patent other antibiotics, silver colloids began to be used less frequently and were forgotten by the mainstream medical community. Perhaps one of the main reasons that colloidal silver faded from use in favor of drugs such as penicillin and tetracycline is money! Almost anyone can produce colloidal silver, but producing antibiotic penicillin at home is an unlikely prospect for most individuals. The pharmaceutical companies promoted their patented drugs, educating doctors in the value of their medicines, while other products (such as colloidal silver) went unnoticed. Thus doctors prescribed those drugs that brought the most money into the medical community.

None of the formerly recognized colloidal silver preparation has been recognized in the U.S.P and N.F. since 1975. The Food and Drug Administration (FDA) now proposes banning over-the-counter colloidal silver products:

> The Food and Drug Administration is proposing to establish that all over-the-counter (OTC) drug products containing colloidal silver ingredients or silver salts for internal or external use are not generally recognized as safe and effective and are misbranded. FDA is issuing this proposal because many products containing colloidal silver ingredients or silver salts are being marketed for numerous serious disease conditions, and FDA is not aware of any substantial scientific evidence that supports the use of OTC colloidal silver ingredients or silver salts for these disease conditions.

Understanding the current FDA policy on colloidal silver and the fact that it was an accepted medical treatment in the recent past, it may be worth considering colloidal silver for use in survival medicine. There are a significant number of testimonials from people who have used colloidal silver in the treatment of injury and illness. I have used colloidal silver and found it effective. It is easy to make and certainly worth further investigation by anyone interested in survival medicine and self-sufficiency.

There are various colloidal-silver generators on the market, but they are all little more than a power supply to run an electric current through silver wires suspended in distilled water. As the current is run through the wires, electrolysis occurs and the positively charged silver ions become suspended in the water. It is this silver-water combination that is used to treat illness and injury.

To make your own colloidal silver generator you'll need three 9-volt batteries, wired in series to produce 27-volts of direct current. From this power source, extend two wires connected to alligator clips. You'll also need two pieces of pure (.999) silver wire. Do not confuse this with sterling silver (.9275) wire; sterling silver contains other metals. Each piece of silver wire should be about 6 inches long. Bend a small hook in the end of each wire, allowing it to be hooked over the rim of an 8-ounce water glass. Connect one alligator clip to each silver wire. The wires should be suspended in the water, but should not touch each other. Within a few minute you will notice the beginning of the reaction as the silver begins to diffuse into the water from the positive electrode. This creates a colloidal silver solution of about 1 part per million for every minute the generator is run (e.g., running the generator for 40 minutes makes a 40-parts-per-million colloidal-silver solution). When making colloidal-silver solution for internal use, you should start with distilled water. (In a wilderness environment distilled water can be obtained by using a solar still.) Colloidal silver intended for external use may be made with only filtered water.

A Final Word

OK, you've finished reading this book. I hope that it has started you thinking and perhaps provided you with a bit of new information. This book (or any book for that matter) can only impart knowledge—it can't give you experience. For that you have to get out into the wilderness and put into practice the things you've read about here.

Start by putting together your GOOD kit and then taking it to the woods over a weekend and putting it to use. What items did you find particularly useful? Were there any items for which you did not find a use? Were there some items not included in your kit that you really needed?

Do you have a wilderness evasion area in mind? Start thinking about this and working on your evasion intelligence package.

Practice your primitive skills. Make a sling and learn to use it. Build a deadfall and be sure you can make it work. Maybe you'll even catch dinner.

Gather some wild plants and prepare them for your next meal. Even if you live in a city, there are likely at least a few areas where you can find a plant or two to prepare. Remember that those dandelions that show up in your lawn are edible.

Finally, make this into a family project. Life does not need to be centered on television and video games. Have your children ever caught a fish? Have you? Is your family self-reliant? If not, now is the time.

Get off of your couch, get into the field, and put it all into practice.

Bibliography and Selected Reading

GENERAL

Angier, Bradford. *Living Off the Country*. Mechanicsburg, Penn.: Stackpole Company, 1956.

Beard, D.C. *Shelters, Shacks, and Shanties*. 1914 (now available from Loompanics).

Benson, Ragnar. *Survival Poaching*. Boulder, Colo.: Paladin Press, 1980.

Davenport, Gregory. *Wilderness Survival*. Mechanicsburg, Penn.: Stackpole Books, 1998.

Fears, J. Wayne. *Complete Book of Outdoor Survival*. Iola, Wisc.: Krause Publications, 1999.

Janowsky, Chris. *Survival*. Boulder, Colo.: Paladin Press, 1989.

Martin, Dale. *Into the Primitive*. Boulder, Colo.: Paladin Press, 1989.

McDougall, Len. *Practical Outdoor Survival*. Guilford, Conn.: Lyons Press, 1992.

Olsen, Larry Dean. *Outdoor Survival Skills*. Provo, Utah: Brigham Young University Press, 1973.

Party, Boston T. *Boston on Surviving Y2K*. Durango, Colo.: Javelin Press, 1998.
Wiseman, John. *SAS Survival Handbook*. London: Collins Harvill, 1986.

COMMUNICATIONS

Ford, Steve. *HAM Radio Made Easy*. Newington, Conn.: ARRL, 1995.
Ford, Steve, editor. *Your VHF Companion*. Newington, Conn.: ARRL, 1992–96.
Hutchinson, Chuck. *ARRL Operating Manual, 7th Ed*. Newington, Conn.: ARRL, 2000.
Ingram, Dave. *Emergency Survival*. Cypress, Calif.: Universal Electronics, 1998.
Kleinschmidt, Kirk. *Stealth Amateur Radio*. Newington, Conn.: ARRL, 1999.
Laster, Clay. *Beginner's Handbook of Amateur Radio*. New York: McGraw–Hill, 2001.

SURVIVAL MEDICINE

Auerbach, Paul S. *Medicine for the Outdoors*. Guilford, Conn.: Lyons Press, 1999.
Benson, Ragnar. *Do-It-Yourself Medicine*. Boulder, Colo.: Paladin Pres, 1997.
Benson, Ragnar. *Survival Nurse*. Boulder, Colo.: Paladin Pres, 2000.
Coffee, Hugh. *Ditch Medicine*. Boulder, Colo.: Paladin Pres, 1993.
Craig, Glen K. *Special Forces Medical Handbook*. Boulder, Colo.: Paladin Pres, 1998.
Forgey, William. *Wilderness Medicine*. ICS Books, Inc., 1994.
Metcalf, Mark. *Colloidal Silver*. Silver Solutions, 1998.
Tilton, Buck. Backcountry First Aid. Guilford, Conn.: Globe Pequot Press, 1998.
Weiss, Eric A. *Wilderness and Travel Medicine*. Adventure Medical Kits, 1997.

BIBLIOGRAPHY AND SELECTED READING

Werner, David. *Where There Is No Doctor*. Berkeley, Calif.: Hesperian, 1997.

Wilkerson, James A. *Medicine for Mountaineering*. Seattle: The Mountaineers, 1992.

Resources

Adventure Medical Kits
P.O. Box 43309
Oakland, CA 94624

Brigade Quartermaster
P.O. Box 100001
Kennesaw, GA 30144–9217

Cabela's
1 Cabela Drive
Sidney, NE 69160

Campmor,
P.O. Box 700-A
Saddle River, NJ 07458–0700

C. Crane Company
558 10th Street
Fortuna, CA 95540

Cheaper Than Dirt
2520 N.E. Loop 820
Fort Worth, TX 76106

China Diesel Imports
15749 Lyons Valley Road
Jamul, CA 91935

Cutlery Shoppe
357 Steelhead Way
Boise, ID 83704

Garmin—GPS
1200 E. 151st Street
Olathe, KS 66026

Magellan—GPS
960 Overland Court
San Dimas, CA 91773

Major Surplus and Survival
435 W. Alondra Boulevard
Gardena, CA 90248

NITRO-PAK
475 W. 910 S. Be Prepared Way
Heber, UT 84032

Recreational Equipment, Inc. (REI)
1700 45th Street,
East Sumner, WA 98390

RESOURCES

Sierra Trading Post
5025 Campstool Road
Cheyenne, WY 82007–1898

Survival Center
P.O. Box 234
McKenna, WA 98558